4 Weeks To Fabulous Challenge

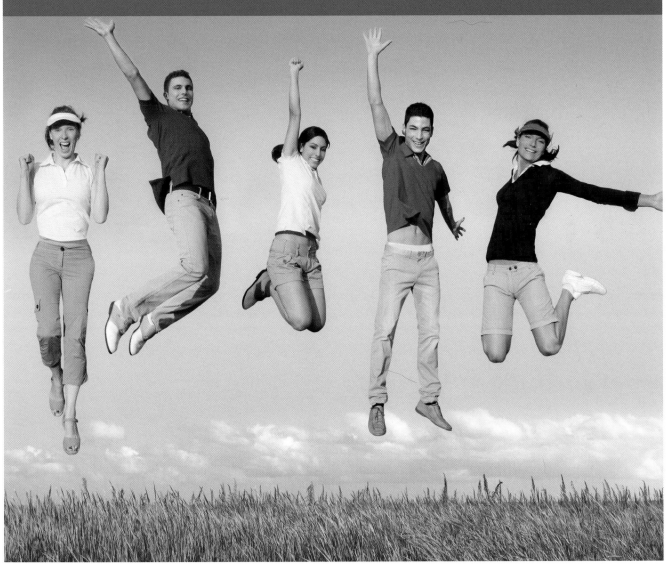

Feel better, look better and live healthier!

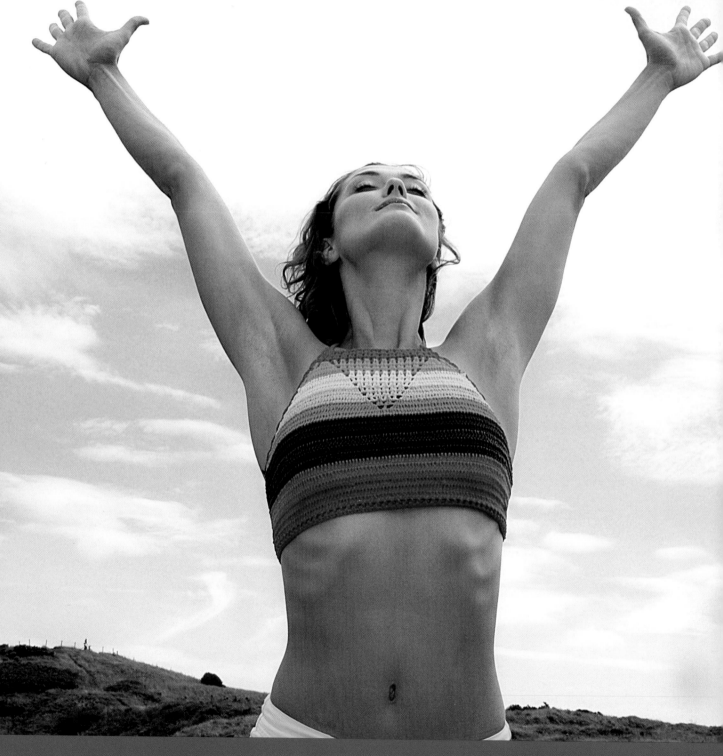

I AM FABULOUS!

I AM FABULOUS!

Contents

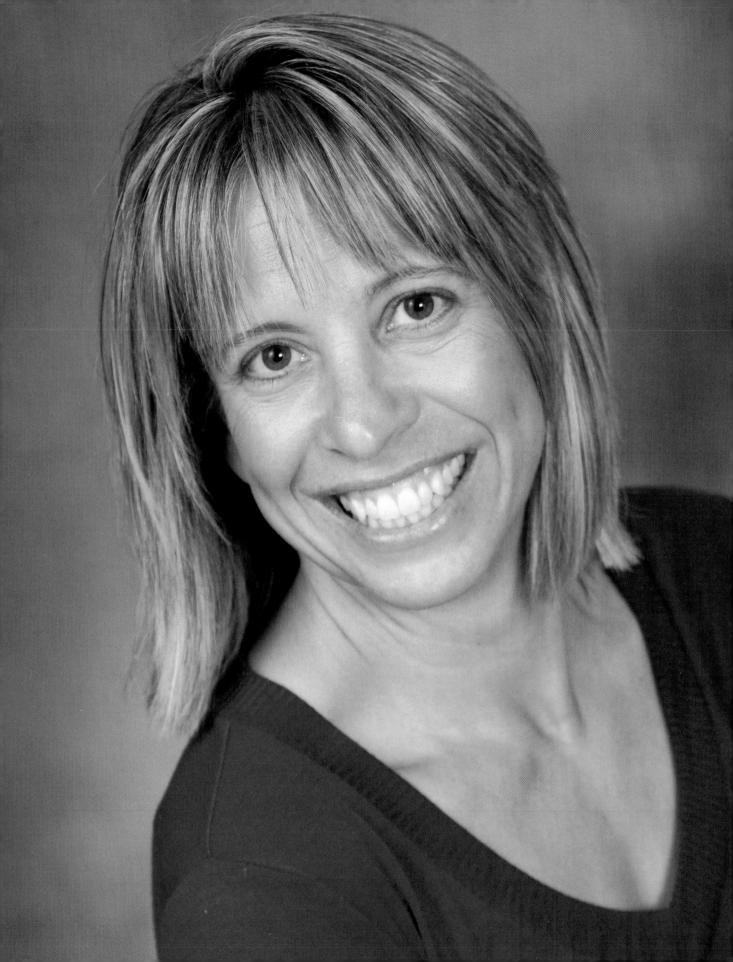

4 Weeks To Fabulous Challenge

The perfect place to start your healthy lifestyle journey!

Dear Reader,

You Can Be Fabulous in 4 Weeks!

A stronger, more resilient body awaits you. Whether you want to lose weight, tone your muscles, or feel more energetic, the 4 Weeks To Fabulous Challenge will help you get there.

Learn how to build a stronger body, fuel your body with wholesome foods, improve your overall health, and overcome personal setbacks. This four-week program can be performed in your own home at a time that best works in your schedule.

Is four weeks long enough to promote change and see results? Absolutely. If you follow this plan closely, you will change unhealthy eating habits to healthy ones—and energize your life. Evidence abounds that the amount and type of exercise you will be doing in the 4 Weeks To Fabulous Challenge reduces the risk in adults of early death, coronary heart disease, stroke, high blood pressure, type 2 diabetes, colon and breast cancer, mental decline, and depression. You will feel stronger, more flexible, and even sleep better at night.

Exercise and sound nutrition are without doubt the most important things you can do to invest in your health. You can expect to spend around thirty dollars for the 4 Weeks fitness equipment--a fitness ball, weights, and a band or tubing—a small investment when you consider the benefits you will receive. Many people have spent that much on vitamins for one month! The truth is many people have an easier time believing in a pill than the capabilities of their own bodies!

Here's to your fabulous self,

Alice Burron

Healthier WY State Wellness Program

Healthier WY would like to ask you this . . .

Are you ready to feel better?

. . . to start something new?

. . . to have an opportunity to improve your overall health?

If the answer is yes then turn the page . . . if the answer is no, turn the page anyway! You will not regret it!!

For more information on the Healthier WY program, contact:

Tammy Till
Wellness Coordinator
State of Wyoming
(307) 777-6716
tammy.till@wyo.gov

www.healthierWY.org

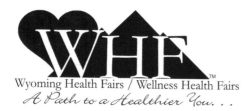

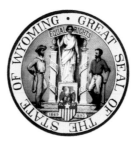

4 Weeks To Fabulous Challenge Quiz

Are *You* Ready For Fabulous?

1. You picked up this book because:
   a) I want to get in shape so that I can look good and feel my best.
   b) I can't seem to gather the motivation to get moving, and hope that maybe this book will be the ticket to looking and feeling better.
   c) It was a total impulse purchase. The cover was so colorful and inspiring I just couldn't resist!

2. How much of yourself are you willing to put into the 4 Weeks To Fabulous Challenge routine?
   a) 90-100% — I'm so ready to feel fabulous!
   b) 80-90% — I'm ready, but expect some obstacles.
   c) 50-70% — My mind says I need to get up but my body wants to finish CSI Miami first.

3. What kind of activities do you like to do most?
   a) Structured, strength-building activities that may be hard but will give me awesome results.
   b) Activities that may be challenging but won't leave me sore in the morning.
   c) Something super-easy that will hopefully give me good results in a short amount of time.

4. How do you prefer to exercise?
   a) With friends or in a group so I have built-in cheerleaders!
   b) With maybe one friend or a spouse, since we want to get in shape together.
   c) Alone. That way no one can tell if I mess up—or maybe skip a couple sit-ups.

5. Are you willing to give up some of your favorite high-fat snacks for things that are a little more nutritious?
   a) Sure. Make over my diet!
   b) It may be hard to give up some of the things I love to eat.
   c) I'm not really that thrilled about giving up my admittedly unhealthy snacks and drinks…are there any tasty and healthy foods out there?

The Results Are In!

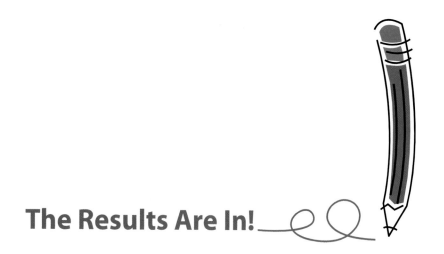

1. Mostly A's
    You're totally ready to get started on the 4 Weeks To Fabulous Challenge Program! It's time to throw out your Twinkies and stock up on fruits and veggies. Get ready to see some results!

2. Mostly B's
    You're fairly ready to get started. It might be helpful to do the program with a friend or spouse for encouragement and motivation. Plus, this way, they'll keep you accountable. If you stick with the program you'll see fabulous results in just four weeks!

3. Mostly C's
    You haven't bought into this whole "exercise" thing yet, but you bought this book anyway. Maybe it was fate, or you knew you needed to get on track. Good for you! It might be difficult to throw out the unhealthy things in your lifestyle, but it will definitely be worth it in the end (and the rear end as well!).

Consider this . . . if you follow this program you will likely lose at least six pounds of body fat and noticeably increase your cardiovascular endurance and strength — enough to run a 5K without injury! Not bad considering all you are doing is giving your body the attention it deserves for four weeks!

4 Weeks To Fabulous Challenge Plan

Make a solid plan! Like anything, preparation is the key to a successful outcome, so before you jump in and start the challenge; let's make sure you've got a solid plan.

Do you have the equipment you need to do the challenge?

Here's your checklist:

- **Weights**
- **Glider/Frisbee**
- **Bands** (light, medium, and heavy)
- **Fitness Ball**

All of this equipment can be purchased on the 2BFIT e-store at **www.2BFIT.net**, or in large retail stores. For additional equipment details, go to Chapter 3: 4 Weeks Physical Activity Plan.

You will also want to be sure to write down your Final Goal at the top of the 4 Weeks Challenge Calendar page on page 5. This will help you remain focused and on track. Make this goal specific and realistic so that you have a greater chance of success. Make sure this is a goal you can measure.

Sample realistic final goals for the 4 Week Challenge:

- **I will lose 1-2 pounds every week of the challenge.**

- **I will lose 0.5% - 1% of body fat by the end of the challenge.**

- **I will drop one pant size by the end of the challenge.**

- **I will gain 1-2 pounds lean mass by the end of the challenge.**

- **I will walk/run a 5K at the end of the challenge.**

After you've set your overall goal, pick a small health habit for each week to accomplish and write each of them down on the bottom half of the 4 Weeks Challenge Calendar. Make sure these habits are realistic and that they will increase your progress toward your Final Goal. Make these goals have bang for their buck — that they will positively impact your health but they're not too difficult or unrealistic. Here are some sample weekly health habits:

- **Only eat 100% whole wheat bread this week.**
- **Always include a source of protein with the carbohydrates with my meals and snacks.**
- **No eating after 7:00 pm this week.**
- **Eat a healthful breakfast every day.**
- **Add one serving of fruit and one serving of vegetables every day.**
- **Eat from home every day.**
- **I will wear my pedometer every day and walk 10,000 steps a day.**

Once you pick a habit for the week, make a check in the box next to "Habit" each day when you accomplish it for the day. If you have a check next to all boxes for each day, all week, then reward yourself (with something that doesn't have calories, or not too many calories). Pick this reward beforehand so that you can anticipate and look forward to it. Continue that health habit throughout the rest of the challenge.

Sample weekly rewards:

- **Go to a movie.**
- **Buy a new pair of athletic shoes.**
- **Make a coffee date with a friend.**
- **Buy a book or magazine.**
- **Buy a new workout outfit.**
- **Get a massage.**
- **Invite some friends over for dinner.**

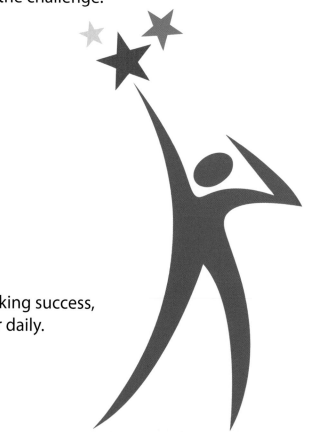

Your 4 Weeks Challenge Calendar is the key to tracking success, so make sure you mark the boxes on your calendar daily.

4 Weeks Challenge Calendar

START DATE: _____   **END DATE:** _____

FINAL GOAL: _____

DAY 1	DAY 2	DAY 3	DAY 4	DAY 5	DAY 6	DAY 7
Pre Assessment						
Week 1 ☐ Exercise ☐ Meals ☐ Habit	☐ Exercise ☐ Meals ☐ Habit	☐ Exercise ☐ Meals ☐ Habit	☐ Exercise ☐ Meals ☐ Habit	☐ Exercise ☐ Meals ☐ Habit	☐ Exercise ☐ Meals ☐ Habit	**Reward** ☐ Exercise ☐ Meals ☐ Habit
Week 2 ☐ Exercise ☐ Meals ☐ Habit	☐ Exercise ☐ Meals ☐ Habit	☐ Exercise ☐ Meals ☐ Habit	☐ Exercise ☐ Meals ☐ Habit	☐ Exercise ☐ Meals ☐ Habit	☐ Exercise ☐ Meals ☐ Habit	**Reward** ☐ Exercise ☐ Meals ☐ Habit
Week 3 ☐ Exercise ☐ Meals ☐ Habit	☐ Exercise ☐ Meals ☐ Habit	☐ Exercise ☐ Meals ☐ Habit	☐ Exercise ☐ Meals ☐ Habit	☐ Exercise ☐ Meals ☐ Habit	☐ Exercise ☐ Meals ☐ Habit	**Reward** ☐ Exercise ☐ Meals ☐ Habit
Week 4 ☐ Exercise ☐ Meals ☐ Habit	☐ Exercise ☐ Meals ☐ Habit	☐ Exercise ☐ Meals ☐ Habit	☐ Exercise ☐ Meals ☐ Habit	☐ Exercise ☐ Meals ☐ Habit	☐ Exercise ☐ Meals ☐ Habit	**Reward** ☐ Exercise ☐ Meals ☐ Habit
Post Assessment						

Exercise: Exercise at least 30 minutes a day for 5 out of 7 days.

Meals: Eat at least 2 servings of fruit and 3 servings of vegetables every day.

Habit: Follow one self-selected healthy habit a week for 5 out of 7 days.

Habit 1: _____

Habit 2: _____

Habit 3: _____

Habit 4: _____

JOURNAL

Success Begins with the Right Attitude

If you have previously struggled to stay with an exercise or diet program, do not skip this chapter. Retraining your brain to think positively toward completing the four-week goal and taking the time to plan around obstacles will bring you to completion and success.

To gain insight into your true purpose and drive behind following the 4 Weeks To Fabulous Challenge program, answer the following questions:

What are my two main reasons for wanting to follow the 4 Weeks To Fabulous Challenge program?

1.

2.

What are the two main reasons holding me back from exercising and eating well now?

1.

2.

4 Weeks To Fabulous Challenge is a stepping-stone and inspiration on your journey to feeling your best.

Now that you have stated clearly why you want to achieve success and what has been holding you back, create a plan to succeed. For example, if your two reasons for wanting to complete 4 Weeks To Fabulous Challenge are to lose weight and feel better and the main reasons you have not until now are because of little time and energy, your action plan may be something like this:

I will make time early in the mornings to exercise while I still have energy, and I will shop on Sundays so that I have meals planned for the week.

What is your action plan? Be sure to write it down, and also verbalize it to others. People who verbalize their intentions to others are 80 percent more likely to achieve them.

My action plan is to . . .

If you are struggling with creating an action plan, read on for tips on how to plan around the obstacles and excuses.

Plan around the obstacles and excuses.

Making time in your day to exercise, shop, and eat right will be critical to a successful 4 Weeks To Fabulous Challenge. The exercises, meals, and even the shopping list are laid out and thought out for you. Now all you have to do is look at your schedule closely and make time for exercise and eating well in your day. Note that this is not the same as finding time in your day, which implies that you have to squeak the 4 Weeks To Fabulous Challenge into your busy schedule, but instead *making* time, which implies that you examine your priorities and identify things that are taking your time that are not moving you in a positive direction, and replacing those things with exercise and eating well.

You cannot fail on your wellness journey. There is no finish line.

Here are some questions to help you decide when in the day and week you will be able to best follow the 4 Weeks plan. I recommend getting out a calendar to mark out your new plans.

1. What day of the week will be the best day for me to grocery shop for the ingredients in the 4 Weeks plan?

2. What time of day is the most convenient time for me to exercise?

3. What time of day do I enjoy exercising the most?

4. Where do I want to exercise?

5. Will an accountability partner help me achieve my 4 Weeks goal?

6. What is my backup plan if my partner bails?

7. What do I foresee as an obstacle (or obstacles) that might keep me from not exercising or eating well?

8. How can I plan around obstacle(s)?

Mark on the calendar your completion date and plan to give yourself a non-food reward when you complete the program. Make a big deal out of the last day!

Replace the excuses with positives.

Let your thoughts about exercise and eating healthily always remain positive. If you relate to any of these excuses, try replacing them with the positive thoughts here.

Eating well and being active—even a little every day—is valuable in fostering continuity. Something is always better than nothing.

To counter this excuse . . .	Use this reasoning . . .
I don't enjoy exercise.	I will redefine the word "exercise" to mean doing a physical activity that I enjoy, and I will look forward to doing it regularly.
Exercise is boring.	I will experiment with different options to make exercise fun such as music and friends and even new exercise clothing.
Being fat runs in my family.	Action and healthful habits can counter genetic tendencies.
I love food so I don't diet.	I can still eat foods I enjoy in moderation.
I don't have the energy to exercise.	If I don't have energy after 15 minutes into the exercises I can always stop.
Healthy food is too expensive.	Healthy food can be less expensive and will keep me from getting sick and spending money on medications.
I don't like to sweat.	I will exercise where it is cool so I don't notice the sweat so much, or choose an activity like swimming or water aerobics.
I don't have time to exercise.	Even short bouts of exercise can make a big difference, so I'll sneak in exercise whenever I can.
I do housework all day so I already exercise.	I do housework all day so I already exercise. While I do housework I will intentionally try to get my heart rate high so I burn more calories and get the most benefit.

Fortunately, attitudes are learned, so we are able to, and should, train ourselves to talk with an optimistic voice instead of a pessimistic one. A good attitude is a choice—so choose to be positive today. Don't let what you can't do interfere with what you can do! (And, don't let perfection be the enemy of good—something is always better than nothing!)

Read the inspirational quotes on the 4 Weeks To Fabulous Challenge workouts to keep you inspired and motivated. Say them throughout the day to stay inspired and exercise your positive attitude (and post them in obvious places).

If you find that you are not ready to embark in a full-fledged weight loss program, make small decisions every day that will get you ready for when you're ready to make a full commitment.

- Carry your groceries in hand-held baskets instead of pushing a cart.

- Do exercises at your desk, which can be found at **www.2BFit.net**

- Stand instead of sit.

- Keep proper posture when sitting and standing.

- Take walks whenever the opportunity arises.

- Jog, instead of walk, from point A to point B.

- Listen to music that you could dance to.

- Sit on an exercise ball instead of a chair.

Be honest — what does completing this program mean to you?

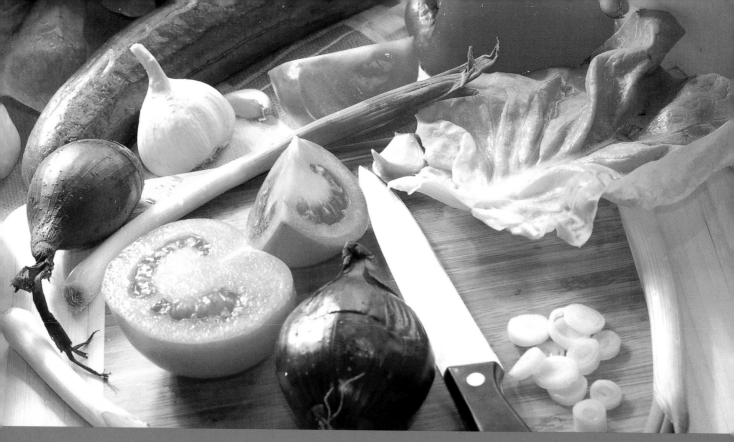

4 Weeks To Fabulous Challenge Nutrition Plan

To accommodate your demanding schedule, the 4 Weeks To Fabulous Challenge Nutrition Plan offers quick and easy meals and recipes designed for busy, health-minded people who desire to:

- Lose weight
- Lower cholesterol
- Control diabetes
- Reduce the risk of cancer
- Increase bone mass
- Improve brain function
- Improve digestive disorders
- Slow the aging process

With so much health information making the headlines, be assured that these recipes are based on recommendations from the American Cancer Society, American Heart Association, and American Diabetes Association and are:

- Low in refined sugars and starches
- Low in total fat
- Low in saturated and trans fats
- Low in cholesterol
- Low in sodium
- High in soluble and insoluble fiber
- High in nutrients, minerals, and phytochemicals (anti-cancer compounds)

The 4 Weeks To Fabulous Challenge menus are meant to be as satisfying as they are good for you. Follow the daily menus or choose from the compilation of meal choices for breakfast, lunch, dinner, and snacks/desserts. A shopping list is included so that you can be sure you have the ingredients you need!

Quality of food is incredibly important, but so is quantity. Unless you know how many calories to eat, you may still gain weight and overeat. Just how many calories should you consume in a day? You can get a pretty good idea how many calories you need a day to maintain your current weight by using the chart below:

Begin each day, first thing, with a glass of water to get your digestive system moving and metabolism started. Continue to sip on water throughout the entire day.

Gender	Age (years)	Sedentary[a]	Moderately Active[b]	Active[c]
Female	4 - 8	1,200	1,400 - 1,600	1,400 - 1,800
	9 - 13	1,600	1,600 - 2,000	1,800 - 2,200
	14 - 18	1,800	2,000	2,400
	19 - 30	2,000	2,000 - 2,200	2,200
	31 - 50	1,800	2,000	2,200
	51+	1,600	1,800	2,000 - 2,200
Male	4 - 8	1,400	1,400 - 1,600	1,600 - 2,000
	9 - 13	1,800	1,800 - 2,200	2,000 - 2,600
	14 - 18	2,200	2,400 - 2,800	2,800 - 3,200
	19 - 30	2,400	2,600 - 2,800	3,000
	31 - 50	2,200	2,400 - 2,600	2,800 - 3,000
	51+	2,000	2,200 - 2,400	2,400 - 2,800

These levels are based on Estimated Energy Requirements (EER) from the Institute of Medicine's *Dietary Reference Intakes Macronutrients* Report, 2002, calculated by gender, age, and activity level for reference-sized individuals.

(a) Sedentary means a lifestyle that includes only the light physical activity associated with typical day-to-day life.

(b) Moderately active means a lifestyle that includes physical activity equivalent to walking about 1.5 to 3 miles per day at 3 to 4 miles per hour, in addition to the light physical activity associated with typical day-to-day life.

(c) Active means a lifestyle that includes physical activity equivalent to walking more than 3 miles per day at 3 to 4 miles per hour, in addition to the light physical activity associated with typical day-to-day life.

If you desire to <u>lose weight</u>, you will want to be thinking in terms of *ENERGY IN* vs *ENERGY OUT*

The same amount of
ENERGY IN (calories consumed) and *ENERGY OUT (calories burned)* over time = <u>weight stays the same</u>

More IN than OUT over time = <u>weight gain</u>

More OUT than IN over time = <u>weight loss</u>

Balancing energy daily is important, but keep it in perspective: you will want to balance energy over time to get to and stay at a healthy weight for the long term. If you indulge and omit activity one day, try to balance out that day with the other days in your week. Try to stay on track more often than not for overall success.

In order to lose weight, create a deficit of 400 to 700 calories from your estimated calories/day needed. This deficit should be from both exercise (burning calories = energy out) and decreasing caloric intake (calories consumed = eating fewer calories). Rapid weight loss (five pounds or more per week) is rarely maintained, and studies show that a balanced approach to weight loss is the most effective.

In the 4 Weeks program, there is a sample menu for each day that contains an average of 1,800 calories, and closely follows the Dietary Guidelines for Americans, which recommends this distribution for the energy nutrients:

- Fat: 20-35% of total calories (average 30%)
- Protein: 10-35% (average 15%)
- Carbohydrates: 45-65% (average 55%)

Use this menu to guide and inspire you to make healthy eating choices, but feel free to use your own favorite healthful recipes. Since every individual's caloric needs are different, you may need to fine-tune your intake to reach your final goal. For example, if you find that you are extremely hungry an hour after dinner, you may want to slightly increase your serving size at dinner the next day, or adjust your servings to include more protein and less carbohydrates. Likewise, if you have not lost weight or inches the first week, you might experiment by decreasing portion sizes, and increasing fiber-rich foods to feel fuller. Keep in mind what a recommended portion size looks like so that you can modify your servings accordingly.

Here are some examples of a single serving size, according to the United States Dietary Association:

- Pasta and rice equal to slightly smaller than a tennis ball
- Meat, fish, or poultry the size of a deck of cards
- Snacks, such as pretzels and chips, the size of a cupped handful
- Potato the size of a computer mouse
- Bagel the size of a hockey puck
- Vegetables or fruit about the size of your fist
- Cheese the size of your thumb

Along with the huge effort you are making to reach your goals, take the next step and cut the processed foods out of your food choices. Eat foods that come straight from the source—the Earth. Fresh or frozen fruits and vegetables (without salt or sugar added), eggs, milk, cheese, unprocessed meats, whole wheat flour, and honey are all one step away from the Earth, not five or six.

Refrain from eating after 7:00 p.m. for best weight loss results. Going to bed slightly hungry will burn off pounds.

Here are some foods that you will want to avoid that could be full of preservatives and void of naturally occurring nutrients:

- soda
- anything with refined and enriched white flour
- chips
- fast foods
- processed meats and cheeses
- candy
- prepackaged cookies
- nutrition drinks/shakes unless made with natural ingredients

If you crave sugar, try these tips:

• keep sweets out of your surroundings;

Here are some tips to remember when you go to the store in order to avoid the processed food trap:

- Avoid high-fructose corn syrup (HFCS) and artificially sweetened foods.

• go for a short walk;

- Avoid foods that say "enriched" or "refined."

- If artificial flavors are added—avoid it.

• chew sugar-free gum;

- If salt was added, try to find the low-salt version—or better yet, the no-salt version.

- Fresh is best.

• drink a glass of lemon water; and

- Look for products with natural ingredients on the label.

- Check labels to ensure that it contains "0" grams of trans fat and is free of "partially hydrogenated oil".

• keep sugary food portions small and take the time to enjoy the experience.

Reading labels before you buy will save you calories, cut out preservatives, and enhance your eating experience. Although everyone eats processed foods at times, the more you avoid them, the faster you will see results toward your goal.

Here's a good rule of thumb . . . *if you can't pronounce a food ingredient, then don't eat it.*

4 Weeks To Fabulous Challenge Menus

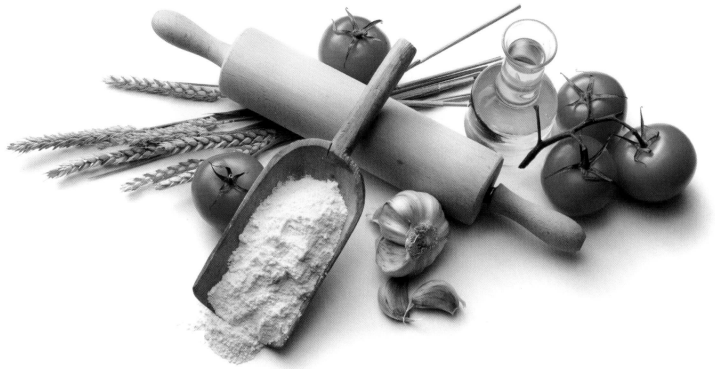

Most of the 4 Weeks To Fabulous Challenge recipes can be prepared in about thirty minutes or less and have few ingredients. Recipes are based on guidelines from the American Heart Association, American Diabetes Association, and American Dietetic Association and are low-sodium, low-fat, simple gourmet style, and easy to follow. Be sure to use the convenient shopping list for once-a-week stocking up. If you have special dietetic needs, be sure to consult with your physician, registered dietitian, or certified diabetes educator who can address your individual needs.

You may want to mix and match breakfasts, lunches, dinners, snacks, and desserts according to your tastes if you prefer one option over the other. Enjoy!

P.S. There are some processed-food options if you can't help but want to satisfy a sweet tooth with something "not-so straight from the Earth." These options are the better of the not-the-best choices, and every once in a while won't make or break your weight loss efforts. Stay on track more often than not and you will achieve weight loss success!

day one

BREAKFAST	1/3 cup granola 1/2 cup fresh berries 1 cup unsweetened or lightly honey-sweetened coffee or tea
SNACK	1 apple *(sliced)* 2 tablespoons peanut butter *(all natural)*
LUNCH	Quesadilla *Spread one 100% whole-wheat tortilla with 1/4 mashed avocado, 1/4 cup nonfat refried beans or black beans and 1/8 cup shredded cheddar cheese. Fold in half and heat quesadilla until cheese melts (either in microwave or on stove top).* 12 tortilla chips *(triangles)* with salsa
SNACK	10 raw or dry-roasted unsalted peanuts, almonds, pecans, walnuts, pistachios or other nuts
DINNER	Tilapia *(3 ounces)* *Drizzle 1 teaspoon olive oil over frozen tilapia fillet and coat fillet sides in a breading made with half Italian bread crumbs, half Parmesan cheese, and a dash of garlic salt. Place on cookie sheet sprayed with cooking spray and broil for 10 minutes or until fillet is golden brown and well cooked.* Couscous *(1 cup)* *Directions are on the package. Use plain couscous, not a flavored mix, made with low-sodium chicken broth and a splash of olive oil. Fab Factoid: Couscous is made from durum wheat, the main ingredient in good-quality pasta!* Salad *1 cup lettuce, 1/4 tomato, 1/4 red bell pepper, 3 halved Kalamata olives, 1 tsp. toasted slivered almonds. Drizzle with olive oil and balsamic vinegar.*
DESSERT *(optional)*	1 cup of sugar-free flavored gelatin *(any fruit flavor)*

Nutrient Analysis for Day 1: 1,632 calories; 76 g protein; 167 g carbohydrates; 78 g fat; 27 g fiber

Fab Factoid: One tablespoon of sugar or sucrose contains 46 calories, while one tablespoon of honey has 65 calories. Though honey may have more calories, it is much sweeter so less is used. Honey also has a healthier Glycemic Index (GI), the measure of impact a food has on the blood-glucose levels. The lower the GI rating, the slower the absorption of sugars into the bloodstream. A lower GI allows for a more gradual and healthier digestive process. Honey also has minerals that table sugar lacks.

day two

BREAKFAST	1 cup oatmeal with non-fat milk 1 tablespoon sliced almonds, chopped pecans or walnuts 1/3 cup fresh berries 1 poached egg
SNACK	1 banana 1 tablespoon almond butter
LUNCH	**Sesame Stir Fry** *Cut four asparagus spears into 2-inch pieces and ½ cup tofu into cubes. Cook on medium high in 1 tablespoon sesame oil. Add ¼ cup water and sprinkle with powdered or freshly minced ginger. Add 1 tablespoon low sodium soy sauce and sprinkle with sesame seeds. Stir to coat.* 3/4 cup fast cooking brown rice
SNACK	2 cups air-popped popcorn lightly sprinkled with salt 1 apple *(sliced)*
DINNER	**Chicken Strips** *(4 ounces - about 4 strips)* *Slice a chicken breast into strips. Dip chicken into a bowl with 1/4 cup olive oil mixed with a dash of Worcestershire sauce. Dredge in a mixture of half bread crumbs and half Parmesan cheese. Place on a cookie sheet sprayed with nonstick cooking spray. Cook at 425 degrees for 20 minutes, or until chicken is sizzling and golden brown. Serve with ketchup or a little honey.* **Wild Rice with Toasted Slivered Almonds** *(3/4 cup)* *Heat 1 tsp. olive oil in a medium pot over medium heat. Add 1 cup wild rice, 2 tbsp. sliced almonds, 1 tbsp. minced garlic, 6 sliced green onions, and 1 tsp. dried thyme. Cook until onions are soft but before garlic is brown. Pour in 2-1/2 cups of fat-free low-sodium chicken broth and bring to a boil. Reduce heat to low, cover with a lid, and let cook for 50 minutes or until rice is tender.* **Steamed Vegetables or small salad with 1 tablespoon oil & vinegar** *1 cup broccoli, asparagus, brussels sprouts or green beans*
DESSERT *(optional)*	1/4 cup fat-free frozen vanilla yogurt with 1/2 cup sliced strawberries

Nutrient Analysis for Day 2: 1,796 calories, 87 g protein, 210 g carbohydrates, 75 g fat, 30 g fiber

Fab Factoid: Although both brown rice and wild rice are good for you because they are low in fat, a good source of fiber, and contain the minerals selenium and manganese, wild rice contains slightly less calories per serving.

day three

BREAKFAST	1 cup shredded wheat cereal with 1 tablespoon slivered almonds 3/4 cup 1% milk 1 sliced banana 1 or 2 cups unsweetened or lightly honey-sweetened coffee or tea
SNACK	Greek-style honey fat- free yogurt (*3 ounces*) 1 tablespoon granola sprinkled on top
LUNCH	Salad with Chicken (*3 ounces*) *2 cup salad greens, 1/4 cup cucumber, 1/8 cup shredded carrots, 1 slice low sodium deli chicken breast, all drizzled with 1 teaspoon olive oil and sprinkled with balsamic vinegar, toasted nuts and Parmesan cheese.* 1 - 100% whole wheat pita
SNACK	1 piece of string cheese
DINNER	Angel Hair Pasta with Shrimp *Sauté in olive oil four sliced green onions, 1 minced garlic clove, 1 tablespoon chopped black olives, and 1 tablespoon sun-dried tomatoes (in olive oil) until onions are soft. Salt and pepper to taste. Add 1/2 cup of uncooked shrimp and heat until pink. Pour over 1 cup cooked angel hair pasta. Sprinkle with 1 tablespoon shredded Parmesan cheese, if desired.* Steamed Broccoli
DESSERT (optional)	Herbal tea such as ginger, lemon, dandelion, or mint tea or sugar-free apple cider hot drink mix

Nutrient Analysis for Day 3: 1,556 calories, 107 g protein, 190 g carbohydrates, 48 g fat, 22 g fiber

Fab Factoid: Shrimp is low in saturated fat. It is also a good source of niacin, iron, phosphorus, and zinc, and a very good source of protein, vitamin B-12, and selenium.

day four

BREAKFAST	1 - 100% whole wheat bagel 1 tablespoon peanut butter *(all natural)* 1 teaspoon low-sugar jelly 1 pear 1 cup 1% milk
SNACK	1 large carrot or 10 baby carrots
LUNCH	Turkey Sandwich *2 slices of 100% whole-wheat bread, 3 ounces thinly sliced lean turkey breast, 1 slice Baby Swiss or Farmer's cheese, 1/4 cup mashed avocado, 1/2 roasted bell pepper, alfalfa sprouts.* Baked chips *(12 chips)*
SNACK	Trail Mix - 1/4 cup
DINNER	Chili - 1-1/2 cup *Fry 1 pound 90% lean hamburger meat (or leaner) sprinkled with 1 tablespoon dried onion flakes, salt, and pepper to taste. Once meat is cooked, drain away fat and then sprinkle with 1 tablespoon chili powder and add 2 cans of low-sodium dark red kidney beans (or see tip below) and one 32-ounce can of crushed tomatoes. Simmer over medium-high heat for 30 minutes. Freeze any leftovers for up to 3 months.* 1 - 100% Whole Wheat Pita
DESSERT *(optional)*	4 vanilla wafers 1/2 cup light sorbet

Nutrient Analysis for Day 4: 1,755 calories, 95 g protein, 238 g carbohydrates, 57 g fat, 33 g fiber

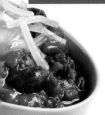

Fab Factoid: To lower the sodium content of canned beans, you can drain and thoroughly rinse them before adding to recipes. Add a little water back to the recipe to make up for drained liquids.

day five

BREAKFAST	1 cup cream of wheat made with skim milk or 1 tablespoon powdered skim milk added after cooking; 1/2 cup fruit; 8-10 walnuts; 1/2 teaspoon brown sugar 1 to 2 cups unsweetened or lightly honey-sweetened coffee or tea
SNACK	1 handful of low-fat, reduced sodium wheat crackers 1/4 cup hummus or 1 piece string cheese
LUNCH	1-1/2 cups chili 5 low sodium saltine crackers
SNACK	2 cups air-popped popcorn, lightly sprinkled with salt
DINNER	**Broiled Salmon** (*3 ounces*) *Coat a salmon filet with 2 tablespoons sesame oil and 2 tablespoons soy sauce, juice from one lemon, and ½ teaspoon ground ginger. Place salmon on a broiling pan sprayed with nonstick spray and broil for 10-15 minutes or until done. Watch closely.* **Brown Rice Pilaf** (*3/4 cup*) *Melt 1 tablespoon butter in a pot and add one bunch of chopped green onion or chives (about 6 stalks). Cook until soft. Add 1 cup brown rice and coat rice with butter. Add 2 cups low-sodium chicken broth and 1 tablespoon dried parsley. Stir, then bring to a boil over high heat. After broth comes to a boil, turn heat to low and let broth simmer at a low boil. Cover with lid and let cook for 40-50 minutes.* **Fruit Salad** *1 diced apple, 1 sliced banana, one 10-ounce can low-sugar mandarin oranges. Sprinkle with cinnamon and mix together.*
DESSERT *(optional)*	1 ounce high cocoa chocolate (*60% or more cocoa*)

Nutrient Analysis for Day 5: 1,756 calories, 95 g protein, 212 g carbohydrates, 76 g fat, 31 g fiber

Fab Cook's Tip: Hummus can be made by processing 2 (15-ounce) cans drained and rinsed chickpeas, 1/2 cup warm water, 3 tablespoons lemon or lime juice, 1 tablespoon tahini (ground sesame paste), 1-1/2 teaspoons ground cumin, 1 tablespoon minced garlic, 1 teaspoon salt, and 2 tablespoons chopped fresh cilantro. Add water if needed. Hummus will keep for several days refrigerated. Tahini can be found next to the peanut butter in the market, or made with 1 cup sesame seeds and 1/3 cup olive oil, processed into a paste.

day six

BREAKFAST	**Veggie Scrambled Eggs** *Sauté 1 tablespoon green onion and 1/2 finally chopped red or orange bell pepper in 1 teaspoon olive oil. Cook until tender, then add 1 whole egg and 1 egg white and mix together.* 1 piece of 100% whole-wheat toast/1 tbsp. light preserves *(low-sugar)* 1 cup grapes 1 cup unsweetened or lightly honey-sweetened coffee or tea
SNACK	1 medium low-fat oatmeal cookie *or* 1 small low-fat bran *or* 1 small whole wheat muffin
LUNCH	**Deli Wrap** *Roll one large 100% whole-wheat tortilla around 4 ounces thinly sliced low-sodium deli turkey breast (or other lean lunch meat), 1/4 cup sprouts or lettuce, 1/4 cup chopped tomato, and 1/4 cup mashed avocado. Slice into quarters.* Baked chips *(12 chips)*
SNACK	Celery stalks *(unlimited)* 2 tablespoons peanut or almond butter *(all natural)*
DINNER	**Meat Patty - 1** *Mix 1 pound 90% lean ground beef (or leaner) with one egg, 2 tablespoons Italian bread crumbs, 1 teaspoon flaked dried onions, 1 teaspoon dried parsley, salt and pepper. Form into a patty and fry in a skillet sprayed with nonstick cooking spray. Cook on medium heat until desired doneness. Drain fat. Serves 4.* **Baby Red Potatoes - 1 cup** *Diced and sautéed in olive oil, salt, pepper, and fresh parsley* **Roasted Asparagus** *Spray a cooking sheet and asparagus with nonstick cooking spray. Sprinkle asparagus with sea salt, pepper, and balsamic vinegar. Broil 5 minutes or until asparagus is tender.*
DESSERT *(optional)*	15 chocolate-covered raisins, blueberries, or cherries

Nutrient Analysis for Day 6: 1,789 calories, 83 g protein, 201 g carbohydrates, 73 g fat, 30 g fiber

Fab Factoid: Avocados are a fruit, not a vegetable. They contain over twenty essential nutrients, are a great source of vitamin K and folate, and high in heart-healthy mono- and polyunsaturated fats.

day seven

BREAKFAST	1- 100% whole wheat English muffin 1 thin slice low fat cheese 1 fried egg in olive oil 1 kiwi fruit 1 cup unsweetened or lightly honey-sweetened coffee or tea
SNACK	2 graham crackers 1 small glass of 1% milk
LUNCH	Greek Salad *Chop 1 tomato, 1/2 bell pepper, and 1/2 cucumber and mix with 1 cup spinach in a bowl with crumbled reduced-fat feta cheese. Drizzle with 2 teaspoons olive oil and 2 tablespoon red wine or balsamic vinegar.* 1 - 100% whole wheat pita
SNACK	1 - 6 oz. container of low-fat cottage cheese *(Optional: sprinkled with slivered almonds and 1/2 cup berries)*
DINNER	Pesto Pasta with Chicken *(1 cup pasta with 3 ounces chicken)* *Cook penne noodles until done. Mix with jarred pesto or make your one. Pesto: blend a cup of basil leaves (fresh spinach can be used for a milder flavor), ¼ cup toasted nuts (pine nuts are best, but any kind works except peanuts), ¼ cup olive oil, and ¼ cup Parmesan cheese, and two cloves of garlic. Add salt to taste.* Chicken *Cut a small chicken breast into thin strips and sauté in a small amount of olive oil. Add salt and pepper taste. Serve on top of pasta.* Sautéed Spinach *Sauté spinach in a small amount of olive oil, minced garlic, pine nuts, salt and pepper*
DESSERT *(optional)*	1 frozen fruit bar or 1/4 cup mixed fruit

Nutrient Analysis for Day 7: 1,640 calories, 88 g protein, 203 g carbohydrates, 61 g fat, 29 g fiber

Fab Factoid: Don't be afraid to eat eggs – they are a good source of protein, riboflavin, vitamin B-12, and phosphorus, and a very good source of selenium. Eggs also contain 210 mg of cholesterol – up to almost your entire allowance of cholesterol for the day which is 300 mg or less. Still, eggs are fine to eat up to four yolks a week.

Breakfast Options

day one
1/3 cup granola
1/2 cup low-fat plain yogurt
1/2 cup fresh berries
1 cup unsweetened or lightly sweetened coffee or tea

day two
1 cup oatmeal made with nonfat milk (1/2 cup old fashioned oats, 1 cup milk)
5 almonds, pecans, or walnuts
1/3 cup fresh berries
1 poached egg

day three
1 cup shredded wheat
3/4 cup 1% milk
1 sliced banana
1 tablespoon slivered almonds
1 to 2 mugs unsweetened or lightly sweetened coffee or tea

day four
1/2 100% whole-wheat bagel
1 tablespoon all-natural peanut butter
1 teaspoon low-sugar jelly
1 pear
1 cup 1% milk

day five
1 cup cream of wheat or rice made with skim milk
1/2 cup fruit, 8-10 walnuts
1/2 teaspoon brown sugar, dash of cinnamon
1 to 2 mugs unsweetened or lightly sweetened coffee or tea

day six
Veggie scrambled eggs
1 piece of 100% whole-wheat toast, spread with 1 tablespoon light preserves
1 cup grapes
1 to 2 mugs unsweetened or lightly sweetened coffee or tea

day seven
One 100% whole wheat English muffin (toasted, no butter) with 1 thin slice low-fat cheese
1 fried egg in olive oil
1 kiwi fruit
1 to 2 mugs unsweetened or lightly sweetened coffee or tea

For recipes see corresponding menu for that day

Lunch Options

day one
Quesadilla
Baked tortilla chips (12 triangles), with salsa if desired

day two
Sesame stir-fry
Fast-cooking brown rice

day three
Salad with chicken
1 - 100% whole-wheat pita

day four
Turkey sandwich
Baked chips (12 chips)

day five
Chili (1-1/2 cups)
5 low-sodium saltine crackers
Tangerine

day six
Deli wrap
Baked chips (12)

day seven
Greek salad
1 - 100% whole-wheat pita

For recipes see corresponding menu for that day

Dinner Options

day one
Baked tilapia
Couscous
Colorful salad

day two
Chicken strips
Wild rice with toasted almonds
Steamed vegetable (broccoli, asparagus, brussels sprouts) or green beans or a small salad

day three
Angel hair pasta with shrimp
Steamed broccoli

day four
Chili
1 - 100% whole wheat pita

day five
Broiled salmon
Brown rice pilaf
Fruit salad
Steamed green beans

day six
Meat patty
Sautéed baby red potatoes
Roasted asparagus

day seven
Pesto pasta
Sautéed chicken
Sautéed spinach

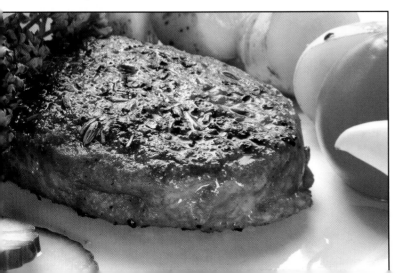

For recipes see corresponding menu for that day

Snacks

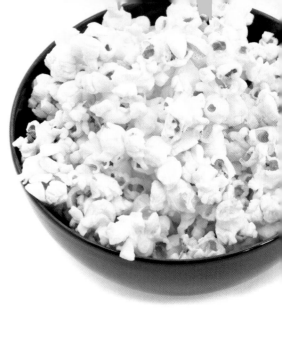

2 cups air-popped popcorn lightly sprinkled with salt

1/2 cup fat-free vanilla yogurt sprinkled with granola

1 small tangerine

1 low-fat mozzarella cheese stick

1 large carrot or 10 baby carrots

1/2 cup trail mix

1 sugar-free frozen fruit bar

1 (12 ounce) skim milk latte

5 whole-wheat crackers with baby Swiss cheese

Celery stalks (unlimited) with 2 tablespoons natural peanut or almond butter

1 sliced apple with 2 tablespoons natural peanut or almond butter

1 small banana with 2 tablespoons natural peanut or almond butter

10 raw or dry-roasted almonds, pecans, walnuts, or pistachios

1 banana with one-inch square of high cocoa chocolate (65% or more cocoa)

1 handful of wheat crackers and 1/4 cup hummus

1 Kashi® TLC® chewy bar

1 hard-boiled egg

1 (6 ounce) container of low-fat cottage cheese
(Optional: sprinkle with slivered almonds and 1/2 cup berries)

1 fruit of any kind

2 graham crackers with a small glass of nonfat milk

1 cup of pretzels

1 medium low-fat oatmeal cookie or bran muffin

1 (12 ounce) nonfat latte

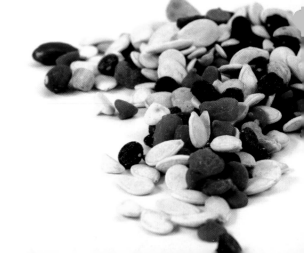

Desserts

Fresh berries and vanilla yogurt

Honeydew, cantaloupe, and watermelon

Plum, peach, apricot or nectarine

Pineapple

1 fruit popsicle

1 cup sugar-free gelatin

1 cup sugar free cider, diet hot chocolate, or hot tea

1 ounce of high cocoa chocolate (60% or more cocoa)

1 small piece maple candy

3 medium meringues

15 dark chocolate-covered raisins, blueberries, or cherries

1 small mint patty

Vanilla Wafers with 1/2 cup light sorbet

1/2 cup fat-free frozen vanilla yogurt with 1/4 cup sliced strawberries

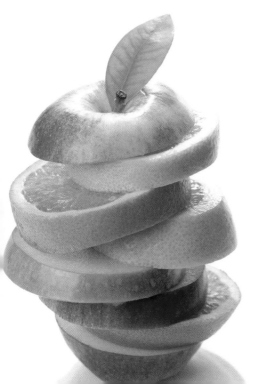

Shopping List

Make shopping easy by using this 4 Weeks To Fabulous Challenge shopping list. While you're in the cupboard, throw or give away any foods that may tempt you take a detour from the 4 Weeks To Fabulous Challenge menu.

Beverages
- [ ] Coffee or tea
- [ ] Sugar-free cider drink mix

Breads
- [ ] Bagels, 100% whole-wheat
- [ ] Bread, 100% whole-wheat
- [ ] English muffins, 100% whole-wheat
- [ ] Muffins, small bran or whole-wheat
- [ ] Oatmeal cookies, small
- [ ] Pita bread, 100% whole-wheat
- [ ] Tortillas, 100% whole-wheat

Canned Goods
- [ ] Bell peppers, roasted
- [ ] Black beans
- [ ] Black olives
- [ ] Chick peas
- [ ] Chicken broth, low-sodium, fat-free
- [ ] Kalamata olives
- [ ] Mandarin oranges, low-sugar
- [ ] Refried beans, non-fat
- [ ] Red kidney beans, low-sodium
- [ ] Sun-dried tomatoes in oil
- [ ] Tomatoes, crushed, 32-ounces

Cereals
- [ ] Cream of wheat
- [ ] Granola
- [ ] Shredded wheat
- [ ] Old-fashioned oatmeal

Dry Goods
- [ ] Brown sugar
- [ ] Couscous
- [ ] Cooking spray
- [ ] Italian bread crumbs
- [ ] Pasta (bowtie, angel hair, fettuccine)

- [ ] Powdered skim milk
- [ ] Rice, basmati and wild
- [ ] Quick cooking brown rice

Eggs & Dairy
- [ ] Butter
- [ ] Cheddar cheese, shredded, 2% milk
- [ ] Cheese, Baby Swiss and/or Farmer's
- [ ] Cottage cheese, low-fat
- [ ] Eggs
- [ ] Feta cheese, reduced-fat
- [ ] Milk, Skim and/or 1%
- [ ] Parmesan cheese
- [ ] String cheese, low-fat
- [ ] Tofu, firm
- [ ] Yogurt, non-fat Greek style, honey flavor
- [ ] Yogurt, plain low-fat

Frozen Foods
- [ ] Frozen fruit bars
- [ ] Sorbet, low-sugar
- [ ] Stir-fry vegetables
- [ ] Vanilla yogurt, fat-free, low-sugar

Fruits & Vegetables
- [ ] Apples
- [ ] Alfalfa or clover sprouts
- [ ] Asparagus
- [ ] Avocado
- [ ] Banana
- [ ] Bell peppers, red, green or orange
- [ ] Berries, fresh or frozen with no sugar added
- [ ] Broccoli
- [ ] Brussels sprouts
- [ ] Carrots
- [ ] Celery
- [ ] Cucumber
- [ ] Garlic

- [ ] Ginger
- [ ] Grapes
- [ ] Green beans
- [ ] Green onions or chives
- [ ] Kiwi
- [ ] Lemon
- [ ] Melon, honeydew, cantaloupe and/or watermelon
- [ ] Onion
- [ ] Parsley
- [ ] Pears
- [ ] Plums, peaches, apricots, pineapple
- [ ] Potatoes, baby red
- [ ] Salad greens (red lettuce, spinach)
- [ ] Tangerines, nectarines, oranges
- [ ] Tomatoes

Peanut Butter & Nuts
- [ ] Almond butter
- [ ] Peanut butter, all-natural (without added sugar, salt, or vegetable oil)
- [ ] Nuts, peanuts, pine nuts, cashews, pistachios, walnuts, pecans, almonds, raw or dry roasted, unsalted, chopped, sliced or whole
- [ ] Sesame seeds, toasted
- [ ] Tahini

Poultry — Beef — Pork
- [ ] Chicken breast
- [ ] Hamburger meat, 90% lean
- [ ] Roast beef, low-sodium, lean, sliced
- [ ] Turkey breast, low-sodium, sliced

Seafood
- [ ] Salmon, wild caught
- [ ] Shrimp
- [ ] Tilapia

Snacks
- [ ] Baked tortilla chips
- [ ] Chocolate, 60% or more cocoa
- [ ] Chocolate mint patty, small

- [ ] Dark chocolate-covered raisins, blueberries, or cherries
- [ ] Gelatin, sugar free, fruit-flavored
- [ ] Graham crackers, low-fat
- [ ] Hummus
- [ ] Kashi® bars
- [ ] Popcorn
- [ ] Pretzels
- [ ] Saltine crackers, low-sodium
- [ ] Trail mix
- [ ] Vanilla wafers
- [ ] Wheat crackers, low-sodium

Spices and Condiments
- [ ] Balsamic vinegar
- [ ] Jelly, low-sugar
- [ ] Cinnamon
- [ ] Chili powder
- [ ] Dried parsley
- [ ] Dried onion flakes
- [ ] Garlic salt
- [ ] Ground ginger
- [ ] Honey
- [ ] Ketchup
- [ ] Maple syrup
- [ ] Oil and vinegar dressing
- [ ] Olive oil
- [ ] Salsa
- [ ] Salt
- [ ] Soy sauce, low sodium
- [ ] Toasted sesame oil
- [ ] Worcestershire sauce

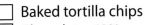

Other:

_____

_____

_____

_____

_____

_____

4 Weeks To Fabulous Challenge Physical Activity Plan

Whatever your goal is — to lose weight, get healthier, or to just feel better — exercise is a critical component. Our bodies were made to move, and the more you move, the better you feel. With just thirty to sixty minutes of activity a day, you will experience strength, energy, and vitality.

This program accommodates two fitness levels: beginner or intermediate. I encourage you to find a fitness level that fits your current fitness status. You may be tempted to jump into the intermediate level without assessing your current fitness level, which you are welcome to do. However, if you become too exhausted or frustrated with the time commitment, you can always move back to the beginner level. The important thing to remember is this—continue the program through week four, whatever level you choose, and don't give up. Starting at the appropriate level, however, will increase your chance of successful completion of the program, and will allow you to achieve the greatest results.

Beginner

If you haven't exercised regularly for a while but are somewhat active, the beginner program is the perfect place to begin. If you're just starting exercising after taking a long break, check with your physician before starting, and, if you are not active at all right now, complete the Start Walking Program in this chapter until you reach week 4, at which time you can begin the 4 Weeks To Fabulous Challenge beginner exercise program. Start the nutritional portion of the program immediately with the Start Walking Program.

Intermediate

If you've been exercising fairly consistently (three times a week for at least two months), you can either start with the Beginner routine (if you feel you need to start a little more conservatively) or go for the Intermediate workout, which requires more endurance and strength but will also give you greater and quicker results.

Once you have completed the 4 Weeks To Fabulous Challenge program, you will be ready to move onto the 4 Weeks to Fantastic Challenge and then the 4 Weeks to Famous Challenge programs — the next two books in this three-book series — so you can attain the most benefit.

Having a partner join you in your 4 week plan makes exercising fun, holds you accountable, and greatly increases your chance of success.

To fully understand and visualize the improvements in your fitness level, I highly recommend that you measure your base fitness level prior to starting. Use the simple fitness tests included in this chapter to assess your cardiovascular fitness and upper body strength. Re-test after four weeks to see improvements.

The Starting Line . . .
Good Things To Know Before You Start The
4 Weeks To Fabulous Challenge Exercise Program

Find your basic fitness level and measurements before embarking on the 4 Weeks To Fabulous Challenge program. Re-test after four weeks, and you will be pleasantly surprised to see improvements! This is a great way to stay encouraged and motivated and to see positive results—on paper and on you!

Before you begin, get your doctor's approval. Your doctor can discuss with you whether it is all right for you to exercise and what can be gained from exercise.

Step Test

Warm up with a five-minute walk. Find a step about twelve inches high (the bottom stair of a staircase works fine, too), and time yourself going up and down that step at a medium and steady pace (96 beats per minute) for exactly three minutes. At the end of three minutes, sit down and find your pulse at your wrist or neck and count beats for one minute.

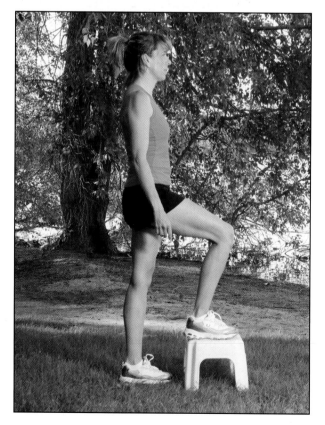
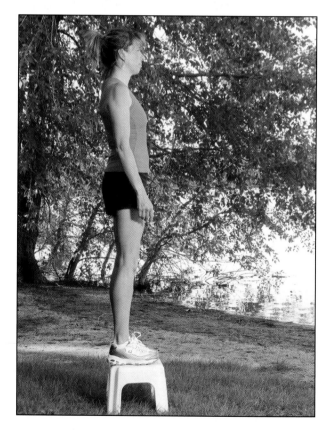

Record your results here, along with the date you took the test.

Before 4 Weeks: Date: _____ Heart Rate: _____

After 4 Weeks: Date: _____ Heart Rate: _____

If you are a man and count over 100 heartbeats, or are a woman and count 110 or more heartbeats, you could use some aerobic conditioning. Follow the Start Walking program in this book to achieve some base fitness before beginning the 4 Weeks Physical Activity Plan.

Push-Ups

Warm up with a five-minute walk, and include stretching and moving your arms. Perform a proper push-up by placing hands on the ground even with your chest and just under the shoulders. Keep your body straight without raising your rear end. Count how many push-ups you can do in one minute. It's OK if you can't continue for a full minute. Record how many you can do until complete exhaustion. Record your results here, along with the date you performed the test.

Before 4 Weeks: Date: _____ # Push-ups: _____

After 4 Weeks: Date: _____ # Push-ups: _____

If you are unable to do a standard push-up at all, don't be discouraged! The 4 Weeks Strength Training program is here to help you to increase your upper body strength.

If you are a man and performed fifteen or fewer properly executed push-ups, or are a woman and performed ten or fewer push-ups, you will benefit greatly from the 4 Weeks To Fabulous Challenge Strength Training program and should see significant improvements in just four weeks. Test after four weeks and record above.

Now it's time to start measuring! Measure the following circumferences with a cloth tape measure. *(Be sure you don't pull the tape measure too tight!)*

Measurement Chart

Before 4 Weeks Date:	*After* 4 Weeks Date:
Weight	Weight
Bust/Chest	Bust/Chest
Waist *(belly button)*	Waist *(belly button)*
Right arm *(largest part)*	Right arm *(largest part)*
Right thigh	Right thigh
Hips *(largest part)*	Hips *(largest part)*
Calf muscle *(largest part)*	Calf muscle *(largest part)*

Start Walking . . .
If you haven't been exercising regularly, to achieve base fitness before beginning the 4 Weeks Physical Activity Plan

Walking is one of the easiest ways to exercise. You can do it almost anywhere and at any time, and it is also inexpensive; all you need are comfortable shoes and clothing. Use this walking program three to five times a week to achieve base fitness before you begin the 4 Weeks To Fabulous Challenge routine.

	Warm Up Time	Fast Walk Time*	Cool Down Time	Total Time
Week 1	Walk slowly - 5 min	Walk briskly - 5 min	Walk slowly - 5 min	15 minutes
Week 2	Walk slowly - 5 min	Walk briskly - 8 min	Walk slowly - 5 min	18 minutes
Week 3	Walk slowly - 5 min	Walk briskly - 11 min	Walk slowly - 5 min	21 minutes
Week 4	Walk slowly - 5 min	Walk briskly - 14 min	Walk slowly - 5 min	24 minutes

Five Minute Stretch Routine

Do the five minute stretch routine, described on the following pages, before warming up or after walking, while the muscles are warm.

Hold each stretch at just the point of slight discomfort, but not pain, for a count of thirty.

Use a support, such as a chair or wall, for balance, if necessary.

Feel free to repeat the stretch routine up to 3-5 times at each session. Breath deeply as you stretch. Stop stretching if you feel pain.

Increase your walking speed to a pace as fast as you can walk.

Hamstring Stretch

- Take a small step forward with your right foot, straighten your right leg, and bend your left knee slightly.

- Lift the toes up on your right foot and lean forward, keeping your back straight and chest forward. You will feel the stretch in your back and the back of your right thigh. For a greater stretch, lift toes up more.

- Hold for a count of ten, then switch legs.

Calf and Hip Stretch

- Take a giant step forward with your left foot.

- Bend your left knee so your shin is vertical but your knee is not extending beyond your toes. Keep your right heel on the ground and your right leg straight behind you.

- Stand tall, extending the top of your head to the sky and keeping your stomach muscles tight. Try not to arch your back. You will feel the stretch in your right calf and hip.

- Hold for a count of ten, then switch legs.

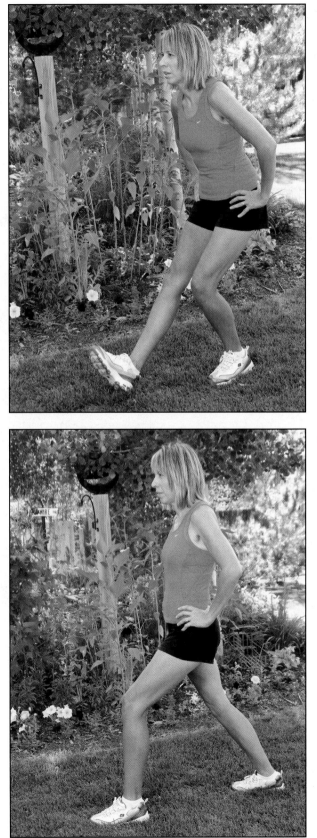

Quad Stretch

- Stand tall, bend your left leg at the knee behind you, and grasp your left toes with your left hand, keeping your left knee pointed toward the ground.

- Pull gently to stretch the front of thigh, hip, and shin. Tilt the pelvis forward and keep both knees together for the greatest stretch.

- Hold for a count of ten, then switch legs.

Shoulder and Back Stretch

- Stand tall, raise your right arm up toward the sky.

- Bend your right elbow so your hand is behind your head.

- Grasp your right elbow with your left hand, and gently pull to the left.

- Hold for a count of ten, then release.

- Switch arms and repeat.

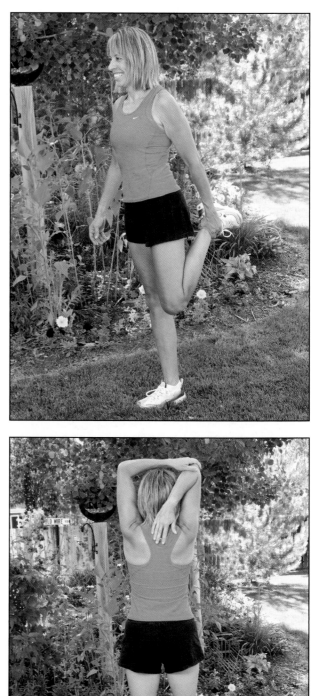

Let's Begin!

Once you are ready to begin, your workout each week will consist of two components . . . **Endurance and Strength Training**

DAY	ACTIVITY
Monday	Endurance and Strength
Tuesday	Endurance
Wednesday	Endurance and Strength
Thursday	Endurance
Friday	Endurance and Strength
Saturday	Endurance
Sunday	Rest

Endurance

At first the sound of the word *endurance* may be intimidating, but it simply means strengthening the heart and lungs. The 4 Weeks To Fabulous Challenge endurance program starts simply with brisk walking every day, but you can use any cardio machine (treadmill, stationary bicycle, stair climber, or elliptical machine) or bicycle, swim, cross-country ski, or do any other aerobic activity in place of walking. Cardio fitness classes — such as spinning, dancing, or aerobics — can also be done in place of your endurance workouts.

The intent is to get your heart rate high enough to cause your heart and lungs to get stronger, while also burning fat. Be sure to do the stretches found in the **Start Walking Program** after your endurance and strength training workouts.

To give you an opportunity to increase cardiovascular fitness and even burn more calories, try the twenty-minute interval workout at the end of this chapter that can be done in addition to or included as a part of the endurance workout. Do not do the interval training workout two days in a row; interval training is intense and without appropriate rest and recovery can increase your risk of injury.

Make it fun — if you don't want to walk, find an activity that you find more enjoyable!

Strength Training

The 4 Weeks To Fabulous Challenge program contains three days a week of a strength training circuit that is performed with no rest time between exercises. Because of this, you will be breathing hard and working the cardiovascular system which will boost caloric expenditure. Because there is no rest time, I highly recommend that you read through the exercises first and make the equipment readily available.

Following the order of exercises is important. By the end of the set you should feel the muscles fatigue and slightly burn. If you do not feel slight discomfort, increase the resistance or weights used.

To add further difficulty, try increasing the repetitions and slowing down the movement. Although the first week the strength training routine may only take around fifteen minutes, weeks 2 through 4 kick it up a notch and will take more time because circuits are repeated.

Warm up for at least five minutes by first walking for a few minutes, then march and add light jumping. Add arms and do some jumping jacks or jump roping. You can also use your endurance workout for the day as your warm-up for the strength training portion.

Always give your body one day in between strength training workouts to recover and avoid injury.

Weight-lifting or cycling gloves are recommended — they protect your hands and increase your grip.

Don't hold your breath when strength training; breathe throughout the movement.

If you feel fatigued before beginning your workout, don't quit but instead start with lighter resistance and repetitions. You may surprise yourself and end up having an awesome workout.

Equipment

For the strength-training workout, you will need the following equipment:

- A five-pound pair of dumbbells; possibly eight and ten-pound dumbbells will be needed as strength gain is achieved

- A glider (large furniture mover, hard plastic Frisbee®, or even disposable Styrofoam® plate also work)

- Resistance bands, light or medium to start, and heavy as needed with strength gain, and door jam holder

- A 55-cm fitness ball if you are 5'0" to 5'6" tall or a 65-cm ball if you are 5'7" to 6'1" tall (a larger ball may be needed if you have long legs for your height or have back problems)

- Sturdy chair

  Gliders, light, medium and heavy bands, weight and balls are available for purchase separately or as a package at . . .

  www.2bfit.net

If you can easily perform more repetitions than what is mentioned in the strength training routine, advance to a heavier weight or heavier resistance band.

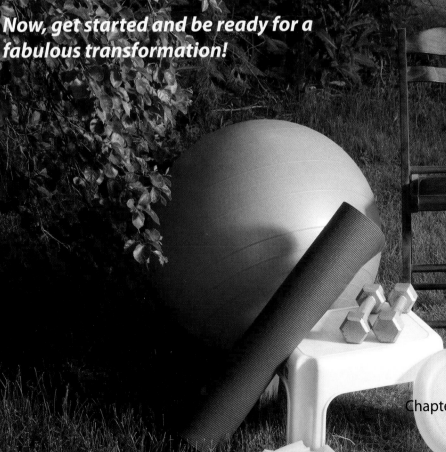

Now, get started and be ready for a fabulous transformation!

The fitness ball will be very firm when properly inflated. Thighs should be close to parallel to the floor when sitting on the ball, although it is acceptable if your hips are slightly higher than your knees.

4 Weeks To Fabulous Challenge Exercise Descriptions

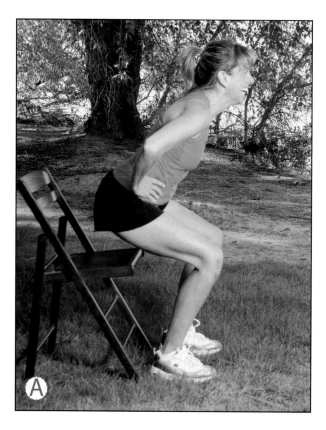

Chair Squat
15 reps

(A)

▶ Stand with your feet shoulder-width apart.

▶ Keeping your back straight, bend from your knees and hips and lower yourself down to a sitting position.

▶ Stop just before your hips contact the chair, holding squat for two seconds before returning to starting position.

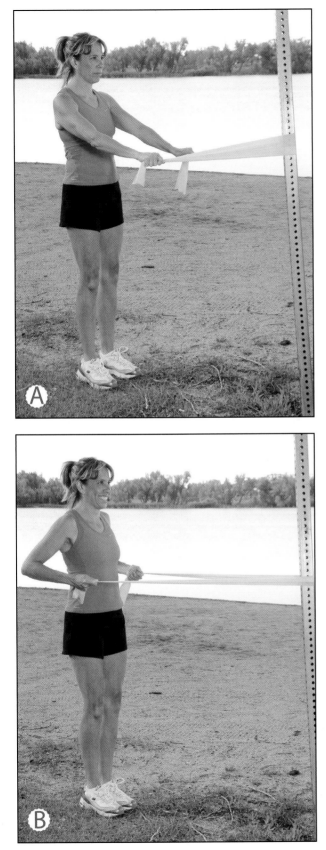

Band Rows
15 reps

A

▶ Wrap band around a sturdy object in front of you, or use a door jam holder, with arms extended in front of you until you feel good resistance from the band.

B

▶ Keeping body tall, slowly bend elbows pulling band toward yourself in a rowing motion while keeping arms close to body.

▶ Keep your shoulders relaxed, squeezing shoulder blades together.

Palms Down Progressing to Palms Up and Palms In

(In subsequent weeks when instructed to turn palms in or up, rotate your hands following each set.)

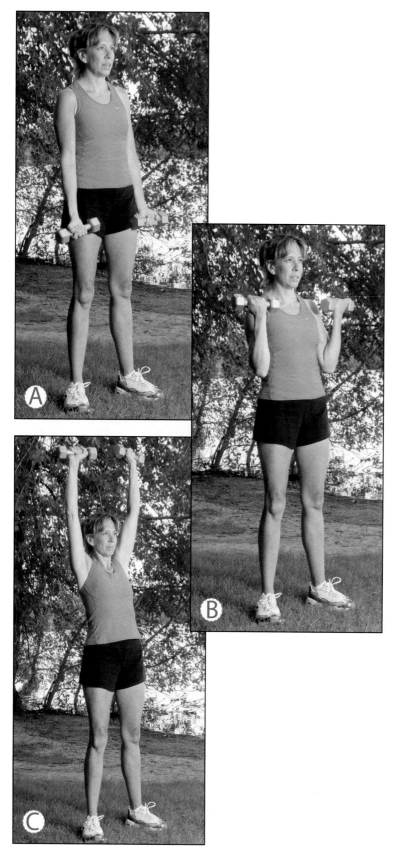

Dumbbell Hammer Curl To Shoulder Press

15 reps

 A

▶ Stand with weights in hands, arms hanging at your sides, palms facing out.

B

▶ Bend your elbows, curling the weights to your shoulders.

 C

▶ Press both weights directly overhead. Lower weights back down to shoulders then down to your sides.

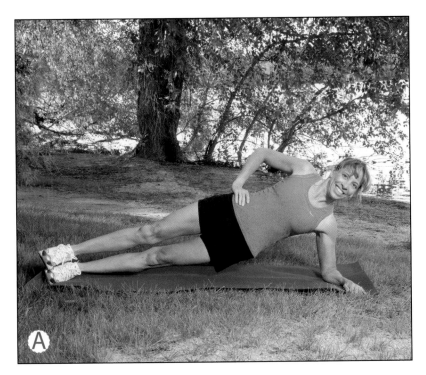

Side Plank on Elbow
15 seconds per side

▶ Lie on your side with your legs straight. Prop yourself up with your left forearm so your body forms a diagonal line, and put your right hand on your hip.

▶ Inhale, brace your abs, and lift your hips. Hold for thirty seconds and maintain steady breathing.

If you can't make thirty seconds, hold for five to ten seconds and rest for five until you've completed thirty seconds in the lifted position.

▶ Repeat on other side.

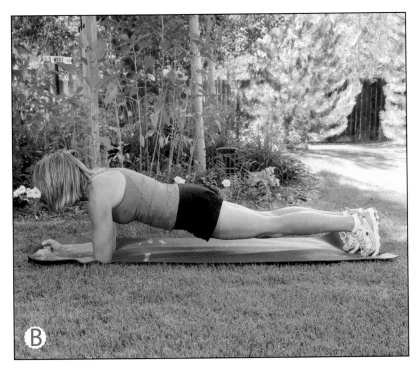

In later weeks, for this exercise you will be moving from a side plank to down plank.

Down Plank
Additional 15 seconds between Side Plank

▶ Position your body face down, balanced on your elbows and toes with your back flat.

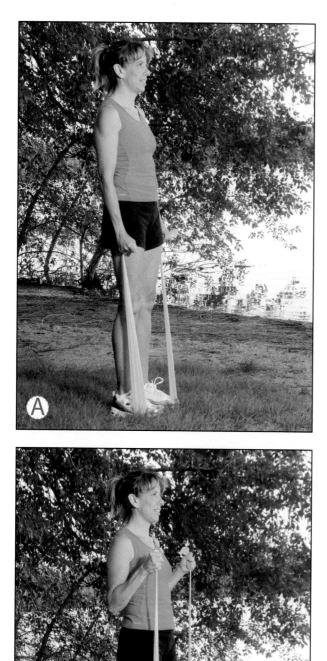

Band Bicep Curls
15 reps

▶ Holding a grip in each hand, stand on the band with both feet.

▶ Palms facing inward, elbows into your sides.

(B)

▶ Bend elbows curling your hands up to your shoulders then slowly return to starting position.

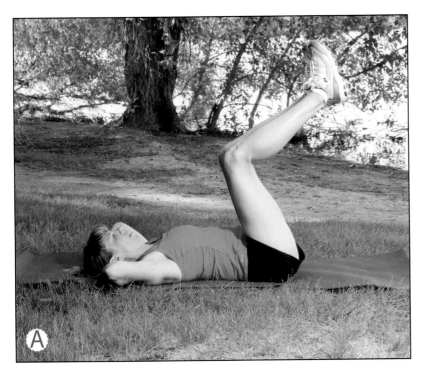

Double Crunch
1 minute

▶ Start by lying on your back, legs extended up toward the ceiling, hands behind your head.

▶ Raise head and upper body in a crunch while raising both legs together and lifting rear off floor.

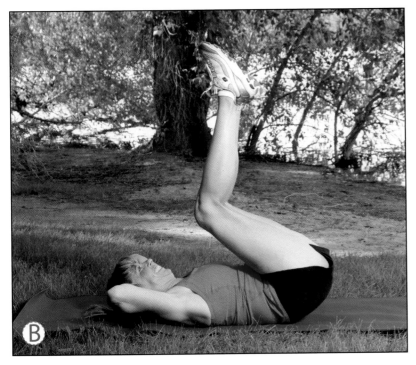

Ⓑ

▶ Hold this crunch and leg lift position for 3 seconds.

▶ Gently lower rear end and legs to the floor and lower upper body at the same time.

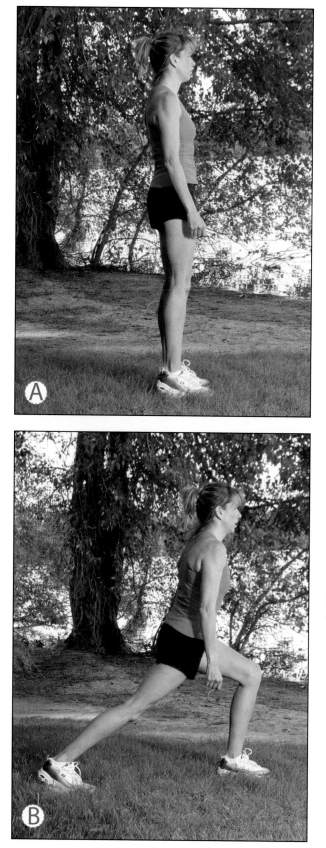

Glider Back Lunge
10 reps per leg

▶ Start on carpet and place glider under your right foot.

B

▶ Balance your weight mostly on your left foot, sliding your right foot and glider back behind you, bending your left knee and lunging.

▶ Return to starting position. Be careful not to overextend by lunging too far back.

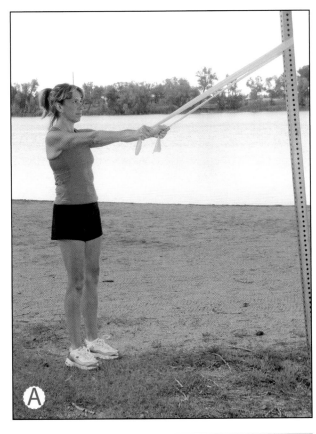

Band Straight Arm Pull Downs
10 reps

A

▶ Wrap band around a post or object at or above eye level.

▶ Holding a handle or band end with each hand, face the object and then step back until you feel some resistance in the band.

▶ Arms should be extended out in front of you.

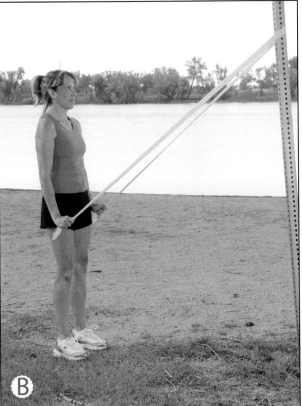

B

▶ Keeping palms down and arms straight, pull the band straight down to your sides, pause at full contraction, then return slowly to start.

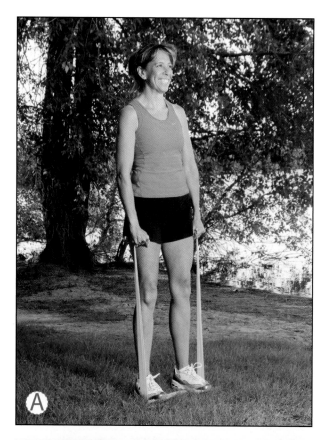

Band Standing Rows
10 reps

▶ Hold a handle or end of band in each hand and step onto the band with both feet shoulder width apart.

▶ Arms are straight down to sides.

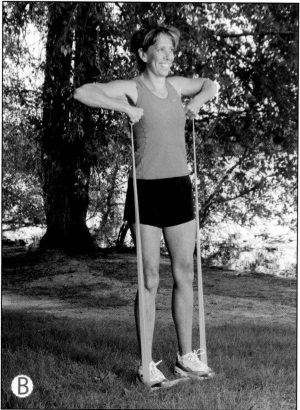

▶ Row your elbows up to shoulder height, contracting your shoulder muscles.

▶ Return to starting position.

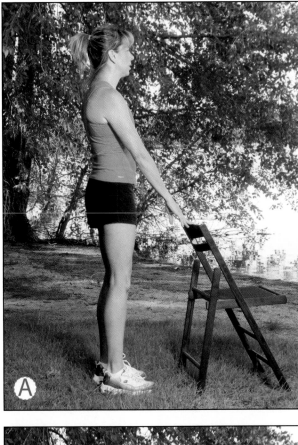

Toe Stands
30 seconds - 1 minute

A

▸ Stand twelve inches away from the back of a chair, with feet about twelve inches apart.

▸ Rest fingertips lightly on chair to help maintain balance as needed.

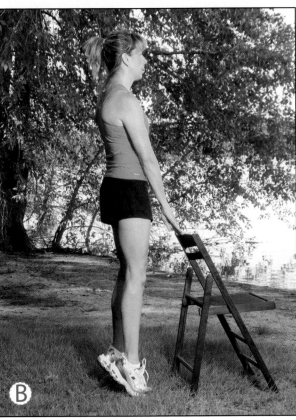

B

▸ Slowly raise yourself as high as possible on the balls of both feet.

▸ Remain on your toes for a count of three, breathing normally.

▸ Slowly lower yourself to starting position.

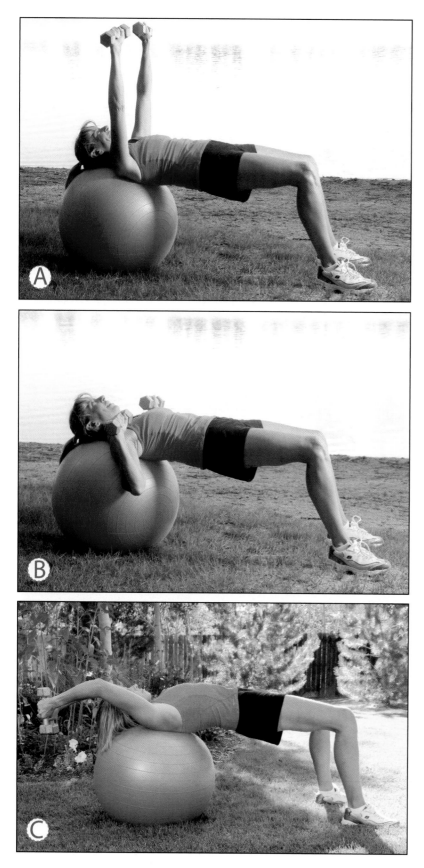

Ball Dumbbell Chest Press

10 - 15 reps

(A)

▶ Lie supine on the ball with head and shoulders supported by the ball. Lift hips so your body forms a tabletop.

▶ Holding a dumbbell in each hand, extend your arms up toward the ceiling with the weights in line with your chest.

(B)

▶ Lower the weights to your chest, allowing your elbows to go out to the side; then extend your arms back up to the start.

In later weeks, as you progress, add the pullovers.

Chest Press with Pullovers

15 reps

(C)

▶ With arms extended up toward the ceiling, palms facing each other, elbows slightly bent, lower weight back over your head, the movement coming from your shoulders, NOT your elbows. Once you have reached a good stretch, slowly return to start.

Axe Chops with Squat

15 reps

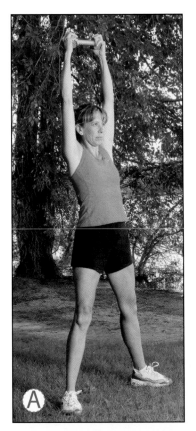

A

▶ Start with feet about hip-width apart, toes pointed straight ahead. Standing tall with dumbbell weight extended overhead in both hands.

B

▶ Lower your body down to a squat, at the same time swinging the weight down between your legs simulating an ax chop.

▶ Keep your back straight and your eyes forward.

C

▶ As you return to the starting position, swing the weight back up overhead.

D

▶ Lean to one side with arms overhead.

▶ Return weight to middle and repeat sequence, alternating sides when performing side-bends.

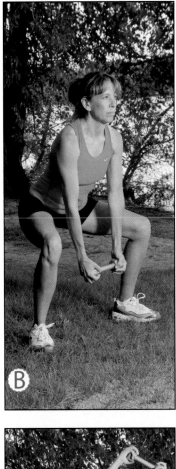

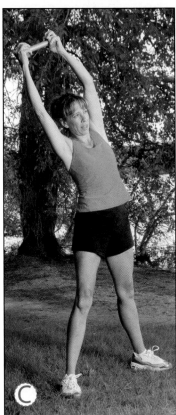

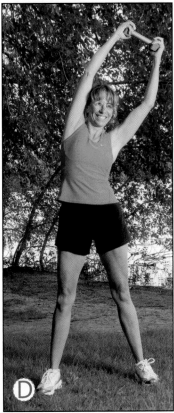

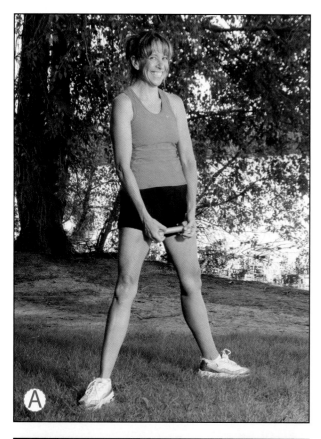

Wide Stance Squat with Dumbbell

15 reps

(A)

▶ Stand with legs more than hip-width apart, toes turned out.

▶ Hold one dumbbell in both hands with the dumbbell in front of you.

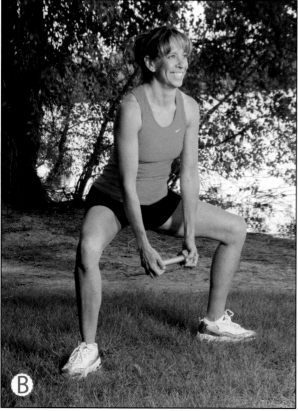

(B)

▶ Keeping your back straight, squat without bending forward.

▶ Pause at the bottom of your squat then return to starting position.

Ball Crunch

15 reps

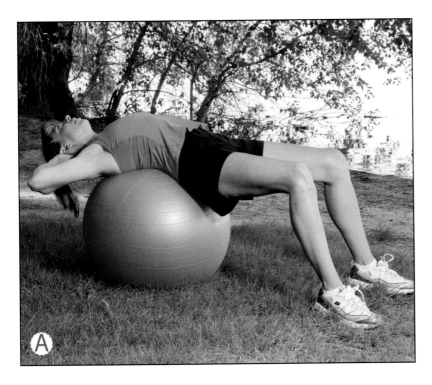

▶ Sit upright on an exercise ball and walk your feet forward, letting the ball roll up on your spine until it is supporting your lower back.

▶ Your head and shoulders are off the ball, knees are in line with ankles, and feet are firmly on the floor.

▶ Place hands behind head and open elbows.

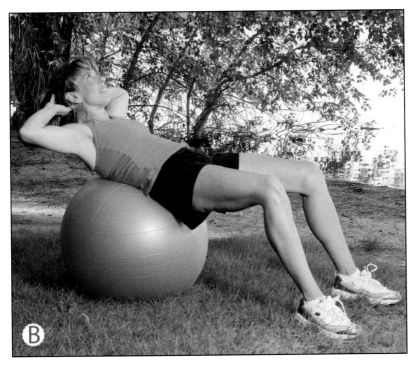

B

▶ Exhale and lift your head and shoulders forward so your rib cage moves closer to your hips, then pause.

▶ Inhale as you lower your head and shoulders back to starting position.

Single Leg Chair Squats

10 - 15 reps

▶ Stand on one foot placing the other foot on a chair behind you.

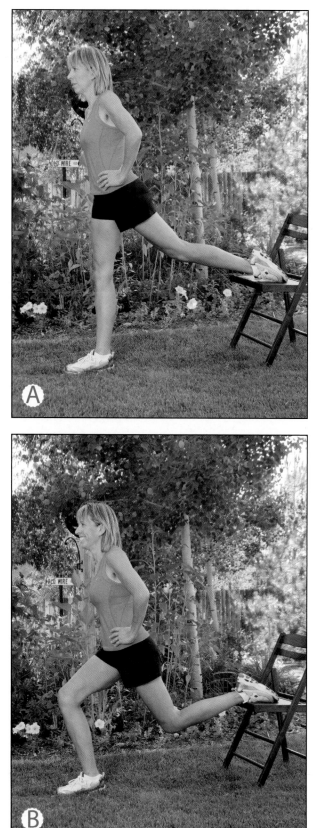

▶ Stand tall, slowly squatting until your thigh is close to or parallel to the floor (being sure the knee of the working leg does not move forward beyond the toe).

▶ Push through the heel of the support leg and return to upright position.

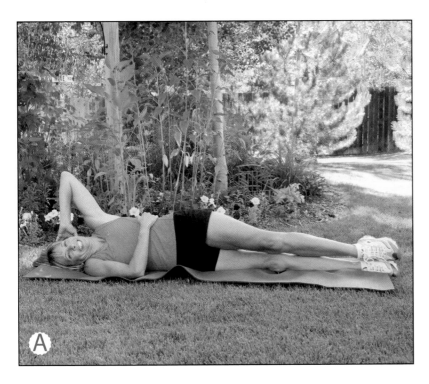

Side Crunch

15 - 20 reps each side

▶ Lie on your right side, legs out straight.

▶ Place your left hand behind your head and your right hand on your left obliques (abdominal muscles).

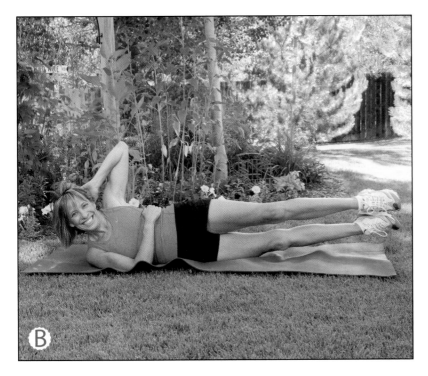

B

▶ Slowly contract your obliques while lifting your left shoulder two to six inches off the ground, being careful not to pull on your head and neck.

▶ Hold for one count and lower.

▶ Repeat on other side.

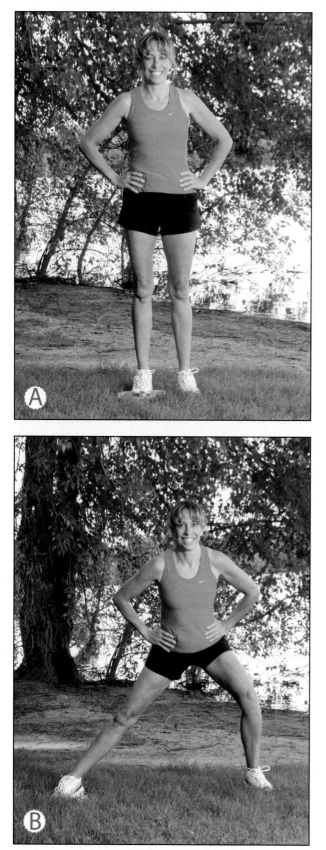

Glider Side Lunge

10 - 15 reps each leg

▶ Start on carpet and place glider under your right foot.

B

▶ Balance your weight mostly on your left foot, sliding your right foot and glider out directly to the side and bending your left knee and lunging to the side.

▶ Return to starting position. Be careful not to overextend by lunging too far to the side.

▶ Repeat with glider under other foot.

4 Weeks To Fabulous Challenge Workout Routine
Week 1 — Beginner

DAY OF WEEK	ENDURANCE	STRENGTH TRAINING *(No rest between exercises)*	TIME/REPS
Monday & Friday *"A man is not old until regrets take place of dreams."* — John Barrymore	10 - 15 minutes fast paced walking *(may be used as a warm up)*	Warm Up Chair Squats Band Rows *(Palms Down)* Dumbbell Hammer Curl to Shoulder Press Side Plank on Elbow Glider Back Lunge Band Straight Arm Pull Downs Band Standing Rows Ball Dumbbell Chest Press Ball Crunch Toe Stands	5 minutes 15 reps 15 reps 15 reps 15 seconds per side 10 reps per leg 10 reps 10 reps 10 reps 15 reps 30 seconds
Tuesday & Thursday	20 - 30 minutes fast paced walking		
Wednesday *"Build your weaknesses until they become your strengths."* — Knute Rockne	10 - 15 minutes fast paced walking *(may be used as a warm up)*	Warm Up Wide Stance Squats with Dumbbells Band Rows *(Palms Down)* Ball Dumbbell Chest Press Band Bicep Curls Side Plank on Elbow Glider Back Lunge Band Standing Rows Band Straight Arm Pull Downs Ball Crunch Toe Stands	5 minutes 15 reps 15 reps 10 reps 15 reps 15 seconds per side 10 reps per leg 10 reps 10 reps 15 reps 30 seconds
Saturday	20 - 30 minutes fast paced walking		
Sunday	Off or light activity		

4 Weeks To Fabulous Challenge Workout Routine
Week 2 — Beginner

*Repeat Strength Training Circuit **TWO TIMES***   **Increase Resistance If Appropriate*

DAY OF WEEK	ENDURANCE	STRENGTH TRAINING * (No rest between exercises)	TIME/REPS **
Monday & Friday *"It is our choices . . . that show what we truly are, far more than our abilities."* — J. K. Rowling	15 - 20 minutes fast paced walking *(may be used as a warm up)*	Warm Up Wide Stance Squats with Dumbbells Band Rows *(Palms Down)* Ball Dumbbell Chest Press Band Bicep Curls Side Plank on Elbow Glider Back Lunge Band Standing Rows Band Straight Arm Pull Downs Ball Crunch Toe Stands	5 minutes 15 reps 15 reps 10 reps 15 reps 15 seconds per side 10 reps per leg 10 reps 10 reps 15 reps 30 seconds
Tuesday & Thursday	25 - 35 minutes fast paced walking		
Wednesday *"We've got two lives. The one we're given and the one that we make."* — Kobe Yamada	15 - 20 minutes fast paced walking *(may be used as a warm up)*	Warm Up Chair Squats Band Rows *(Palms Down)* Dumbbell Hammer Curl to Shoulder Press Side Plank on Elbow Glider Back Lunge Band Straight Arm Pull Downs Band Standing Rows Ball Dumbbell Chest Press Ball Crunch Toe Stands	5 minutes 15 reps 15 reps 15 reps 15 seconds per side 10 reps per leg 10 reps 10 reps 10 reps 15 reps 45 seconds
Saturday	25 - 35 minutes fast paced walking		
Sunday	Off or light activity		

4 Weeks To Fabulous Challenge Workout Routine
Week 3 — Beginner

*Repeat Strength Training Circuit **TWO TIMES**   **Increase Resistance If Appropriate

DAY OF WEEK	ENDURANCE	STRENGTH TRAINING * (No rest between exercises)	TIME/REPS **
Monday & Friday *"The race goes not always to the swift, but to those who keep on running."* *—Unknown*	20 - 25 minutes fast paced walking *(may be used as a warm up)*	Warm Up Chair Squats Band Rows *(Palms Down to Palms Up)* Dumbbell Hammer Curl to Shoulder Press Side Plank on Elbow Glider Back Lunge Band Straight Arm Pull Downs Band Standing Rows Ball Dumbbell Chest Press Ball Crunch Toe Stands	5 minutes 15 reps 15 reps each 15 reps 30 seconds per side 15 reps per leg 15 reps 15 reps 15 reps 15 reps 1 minute
Tuesday & Thursday	35 - 45 minutes fast paced walking *include interval workout*		
Wednesday *"We cannot direct the wind, but we can adjust the sails."* *— Bertha Calloway*	10 - 15 minutes fast paced walking *(may be used as a warm up)*	Warm Up Wide Stance Squats with Dumbbells Band Rows *(Palms Down)* Ball Dumbbell Chest Press Band Bicep Curls Side Plank on Elbow Glider Back Lunge Band Standing Rows Band Straight Arm Pull Downs Ball Crunch Toe Stands	5 minutes 15 reps 15 reps 10 reps 15 reps 30 seconds per side 10 reps per leg 10 reps 10 reps 15 reps 30 seconds
Saturday	35 - 45 minutes fast paced walking *include interval workout*		
Sunday	Off or light activity		

4 Weeks To Fabulous Challenge Workout Routine
Week 4 — Beginner

*Repeat Strength Training Circuit **THREE TIMES***   **Increase Resistance If Appropriate

DAY OF WEEK	ENDURANCE	STRENGTH TRAINING * (No rest between exercises)	TIME/REPS **
Monday & Friday *"The less tension and effort, the faster and more powerful you will be."* *—Bruce Lee*	20 - 25 minutes fast paced walking *(may be used as a warm up)*	Warm Up Wide Stance Squats with Dumbbells Band Rows *(Palms Down to Palms Up)* Ball Dumbbell Chest Press Band Bicep Curls Side Plank on Elbow to Down Plank Glider Back Lunge Band Standing Rows Band Straight Arm Pull Downs Ball Crunch Toe Stands	5 minutes 15 reps 15 reps 10 reps 15 reps 30 seconds per side 15 reps per leg 15 reps 15 reps 15 reps 1 minute
Tuesday & Thursday	45 - 55 minutes fast paced walking *include interval workout*		
Wednesday *"Ninety percent of the game is half mental."* *— Yogi Berra*	20 - 25 minutes fast paced walking *(may be used as a warm up)*	Warm Up Chair Squats Band Rows *(Palms Down to Palms Up)* Dumbbell Hammer Curl to Shoulder Press Side Plank on Elbow to Down Plank Glider Back Lunge Band Straight Arm Pull Downs Band Standing Rows Ball Dumbbell Chest Press Ball Crunch Toe Stands	5 minutes 15 reps 15 reps each 15 reps 30 seconds per side 15 reps per leg 15 reps 15 reps 15 reps 15 reps 1 minute
Saturday	45 - 55 minutes fast paced walking *include interval workout*		
Sunday	Off or light activity		

4 Weeks To Fabulous Challenge Workout Routine
Week 1 — Intermediate

DAY OF WEEK	ENDURANCE	STRENGTH TRAINING (No rest between exercises)	TIME/REPS
Monday & Friday *"If you don't like something, change it; if you can't change it, change the way you think about it."* — Mary Engelbreit	15 - 20 minutes fast paced walking *(may be used as a warm up)*	Warm Up Axe Chops with Squats Band Rows *(Palms Down to Palm Up)* Ball Dumbbell Chest Press Side Plank on Elbow Glider Back Lunge Toe Stands Band Straight Arm Pull Downs Band Standing Rows Dumbbell Hammer Curl to Shoulder Press Ball Crunch	5 minutes 15 reps 15 reps each 15 reps 30 seconds per side 10 reps per leg 45 seconds 15 reps 15 reps 15 reps 1 minute
Tuesday & Thursday	25 - 30 minutes fast paced walking		
Wednesday *"We are what we repeatedly do. Excellence, then, is not an act, but a habit."* — Aristotle	15 - 20 minutes fast paced walking *(may be used as a warm up)*	Warm Up Single Leg Chair Squats Band Straight Arm Pull Downs Ball Dumbbell Chest Press Side Crunch Glider Side Lunge Toe Stands Band Rows *(Palms Down to Palms Up)* Band Standing Rows Dumbbell Bicep Curls to Shoulder Press Double Crunch	5 minutes 10 reps 15 reps 15 reps 15 reps per side 10 reps per leg 45 seconds 15 reps each 15 reps 15 reps 1 minute
Saturday	25 - 35 minutes fast paced walking		
Sunday	Off or light activity		

4 Weeks To Fabulous Challenge Workout Routine
Week 2 — Intermediate
**Increase Resistance If Appropriate

DAY OF WEEK	ENDURANCE	STRENGTH TRAINING (No rest between exercises)	TIME/REPS **
Monday & Friday *"Be not afraid of going slowly; be afraid only of standing still."* — *Chinese Proverb*	20 - 25 minutes fast paced walking *(may be used as a warm up)*	Warm Up Single Leg Chair Squats Band Straight Arm Pull Downs Ball Dumbbell Chest Press Side Crunch Glider Side Lunge Toe Stands Band Rows *(Palms Down to Palms Up)* Band Standing Rows Dumbbell Bicep Curls to Shoulder Press Double Crunch	5 minutes 12 reps 15 reps 15 reps 15 reps per side 12 reps per leg 1 minute 15 reps each 15 reps 15 reps 1 minute
Tuesday & Thursday	35 - 40 minutes fast paced walking		
Wednesday *"Our actions are the spring of our happiness or misery."* — *Phillip Skelton*	20 - 25 minutes fast paced walking *(may be used as a warm up)*	Warm Up Axe Chops with Squats Band Rows *(Palms Down to Palm Up)* Ball Dumbbell Chest Press Side Plank on Elbow Glider Back Lunge Toe Stands Band Straight Arm Pull Downs Band Standing Rows Dumbbell Hammer Curl to Shoulder Press Ball Crunch	5 minutes 15 reps 15 reps each 15 reps 30 seconds per side 12 reps per leg 45 seconds 15 reps 15 reps 15 reps 1 minute
Saturday	35 - 40 minutes fast paced walking		
Sunday	Off or light activity		

4 Weeks To Fabulous Challenge Workout Routine
Week 3 — Intermediate

*Repeat Strength Training Circuit **TWO TIMES***   **Increase Resistance If Appropriate

DAY OF WEEK	ENDURANCE	STRENGTH TRAINING * (No rest between exercises)	TIME/REPS **
Monday & Friday *"It takes courage to grow up and turn out to be who you really are."* — E. E. Cummings	15 - 20 minutes fast paced walking *(may be used as a warm up)*	Warm Up Axe Chops with Squats Weight/Side Bends Band Rows *(Palms Down to Palm Up)* Ball Dumbbell Chest Press to Pullovers Side Plank on Elbow to Down Plank Glider Back Lunge Toe Stands Band Straight Arm Pull Downs Band Standing Rows Dumbbell Hammer Curl to Shoulder Press Ball Crunch	5 minutes 15 reps 15 reps each 15 reps 30 seconds per side 15 reps per leg 1 minute 20 reps 20 reps 15 reps 1 minute
Tuesday & Thursday	25 - 30 minutes fast paced walking		
Wednesday *"Sometimes you have to get worse before you get better."* — Tom Watson	15 - 20 minutes fast paced walking *(may be used as a warm up)*	Warm Up Single Leg Chair Squats Band Straight Arm Pull Downs Ball Dumbbell Chest Press Side Crunch Glider Side Lunge Toe Stands Band Rows *(Palms Down to Palms Up)* Band Standing Rows Dumbbell Hammer Curl to Shoulder Press Double Crunch	5 minutes 15 reps 20 reps 15 reps 15 reps per side 15 reps per leg 1 minute 15 reps each 20 reps 15 reps 1 minute
Saturday	25 - 35 minutes fast paced walking		
Sunday	Off or light activity		

4 Weeks To Fabulous Challenge Workout Routine
Week 4 — Intermediate

*Repeat Strength Training Circuit **THREE TIMES**   **Increase Resistance If Appropriate

DAY OF WEEK	ENDURANCE	STRENGTH TRAINING * (No rest between exercises)	TIME/REPS **
Monday & Friday *"A man who wants something will find a way; a man who doesn't will find an excuse."* — Stephan Dolley Jr.	30 - 35 minutes fast paced walking *(may be used as a warm up)*	Warm Up Single Leg Chair Squats Band Straight Arm Pull Downs Ball Dumbbell Chest Press Side Crunch Glider Side Lunge Toe Stands Band Rows *(Palms Down to Palms Up)* Band Standing Rows Dumbbell Hammer Curl to Shoulder Press Reverse Crunch	5 minutes 15 reps 20 reps 15 reps 20 reps per side 15 reps per leg 1 minute 15 reps each 20 reps 15 reps 1 minute
Tuesday & Thursday	45 - 55 minutes fast paced walking		
Wednesday *"Our actions are the spring of our happiness or misery."* — Phillip Skelton	30 - 35 minutes fast paced walking *(may be used as a warm up)*	Warm Up Axe Chops with Squats Weight/Side Bends Band Rows *(Palms Down to Palm Up)* Ball Dumbbell Chest Press to Pullovers Side Plank on Elbows to Down Plank Glider Back Lunge Toe Stands Band Straight Arm Pull Downs Band Standing Rows Dumbbell Hammer Curl to Shoulder Press Ball Crunch	5 minutes 15 reps 15 reps each 15 reps 45 seconds per side 15 reps per leg 1 minute 20 reps 20 reps 15 reps 1 minute
Saturday	55 - 60 minutes fast paced walking		
Sunday	Off or light activity		

Supercharge Your Workout...with Interval Training

Interval training is an exercise technique used by elite athletes to boost speed, power and endurance. Establishing strong base-level fitness is a good idea before adding interval training to your endurance workout. If your body is ready for more challenge, add this routine to boost heart and lung strength and weight loss results.

Interval training keeps your heart rate at a higher level than exercising at a steady pace—and pushes your body to get stronger. Your body will not be anticipating the intensity, so it will burn more calories not only during the higher intensity bout—but also during the rest periods in between.

You can do interval training on a bike, any cardio machine, walking, running, or even in a pool. Try this program two to three times a week to shake up your routine, lose weight, add speed and power to your sport, or just to beat boredom. Don't forget to warm up well prior to beginning, and stretch after the workout.

20 Minute Interval Program

* Rate your intensity on a scale of 1 to 10.

1 — is very, very light.

2-3 — is light.

5-6 — is somewhat hard but still enables you to talk fairly comfortably.

7-8 — is hard.

9 — is very, very hard.

10 — is total exhaustion.

MINUTES	INTENSITY *
1:00 - 4:00	3-5
4:00 - 4:30	6
4:30 - 6:00	4
6:00 - 6:30	7
6:30 - 8:00	4
8:00 - 8:30	8
8:30 - 10:00	5
10: 00 - 10:30	9
10:30 - 12:00	5
12:00 - 12:30	8
12:30 - 14:00	5
14:00 - 14:30	7
14:30 - 16:00	4
16:00 - 16:30	6
16:30 - 20:00	3-4

Resources

and further reading for sound lifestyle guidelines and information.

American Cancer Society
www.cancer.org

American College of Sports Medicine
www.acsm.org

American Council on Exercise
www.acefitness.org

American Diabetes Association
www.diabetes.org

American Dietetic Association
www.eatright.org

American Heart Association
www.heart.org

Center for Disease Control and Prevention
www.fruitsandveggiesmatter.gov

National Strength and Conditioning Association
www.nsca-lift.org

United States Department of Agriculture
www.usda.gov
www.nutrition.gov

Wyoming Health Fairs
www.wyominghealthfairs.com

**Visit Alice's blog at . . . www.2BFIT.net
for fitness products, books, healthy tips and health articles.**

About The Author
Alice Burron

Fifteen years experience getting people motivated to live healthy lifestyles has established Alice as a fitness and wellness expert go-to for interviews by national publications and as a national presenter. After having four children, Alice has been able to successfully lose excess pregnancy weight and return to her pre-pregnancy weight and stay there, and she attributes her success to sound healthy lifestyle principles she presents in this book.

Alice earned a Master's Degree in Physical Education with an emphasis in Exercise Physiology from the University of Wyoming and is an American Council on Exercise (ACE) Certified Personal Trainer and Weight Management Consultant. She has been interviewed as an ACE national spokesperson by magazines and online publications. She is also a fitness expert for several online publications.

Visit her blog at
www.2BFIT.net
for healthy tips and articles.
Her second and third
books that follow
*4 Weeks To Fabulous
Challenge, 4 Weeks To
Fantastic Challenge* and
*4 Weeks To Famous
Challenge*, are scheduled
for release in 2012.

*Speaking opportunities,
individual and corporate
wellness consultations,
additional books and bulk
order discounts can
be requested at*
contact@2BFIT.net

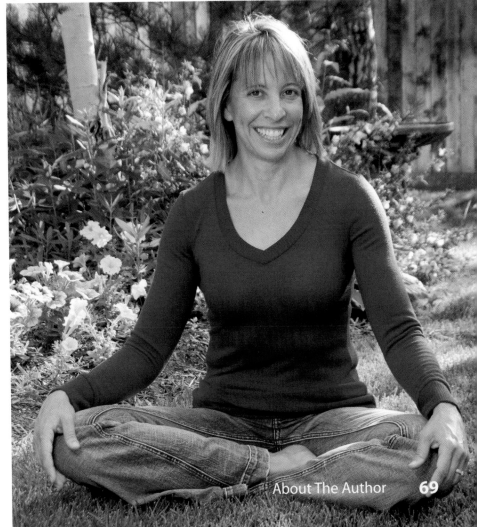

Acknowledgements

"The Lord will continually guide you; He will satisfy your needs . . . and will strengthen your frame. You will be like a well-watered garden, like a spring whose waters never fail."

Isaiah 58:11

My family rocks. Words can't express how much I love them all: my amazing and supportive husband, the best four children anyone could ever wish for, and my parents who love me and support everything I do.

Thank you to all who contributed or supported any part of this book and fitness program.

In particular I'd like to thank Mary Bushkuhl with Mary's Fitness *(www.wyogetfit.com)* for her contribution to the physical activity plan, Val Rothwell with Val Rothwell Photography *(www. valrothwellphoto.com)* for the photographs and Janelle Shields with Phantasm Graphics *(www.phantasmgraphics.com)* for the redesign, and those that tested the program and gave me valuable feedback.

Lastly, thank YOU for embarking on a healthy lifestyle journey! Wellness journeys never end, but they are one of the most rewarding and gratifying experiences you will ever encounter.

My best to you . . .

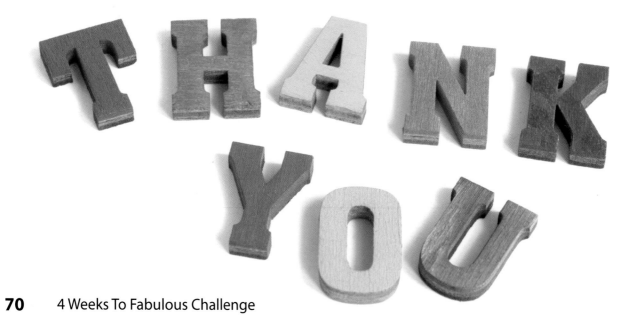